AF256415

Margaret S. Winchester • Caprice A. Knapp
Rhonda BeLue

Editors

Global Health Collaboration

Challenges and Lessons

Editors
Margaret S. Winchester
Department of Health Policy
and Administration
Pennsylvania State University
University Park, PA, USA

Caprice A. Knapp
Department of Health Policy
and Administration
Pennsylvania State University
University Park, PA, USA

Rhonda BeLue
Department of Health Management
and Policy
Saint Louis University
St. Louis, MO, USA

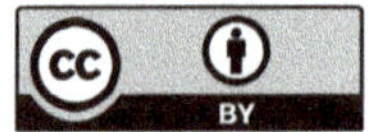

https://doi.org/10.1007/978-3-319-77685-9

Acknowledgments

The Pan Institution Network for Global Health (PINGH) is more than the sum of its parts. We are deeply thankful to each of the members and their involvement, in all of its forms. Our institutional partners include faculty members and supportive administrators at The Pennsylvania State University, University of Freiburg, University of Cape Town, Savitribai Phule Pune University, University of Limpopo, University of the West Indies, and Mountcrest University College.

The following offices at The Pennsylvania State University were responsible for the initial connections and resources that brought us together: Global Programs, the College of Health and Human Development, and Office of the Vice President for Research. We also thank the University of West Indies at Cave Hill Campus for hosting a PINGH writing intensive workshop in August 2017 to give us the space to work collaboratively and refine our writing together. Diane Farley has provided cheerful and invaluable administrative support in preparation of the manuscript. We thank Dr. Shalini Poorasingh for thoughtful comments on all the chapters.

Contents

The original version of this book was revised. An erratum to this book can be found at
https://doi.org/10.1007/978-3-319-77685-9_10

Chapter 1
Building Sustainable Networks: Introducing the Pan Institution Network for Global Health

Margaret S. Winchester, Caprice Knapp, and Rhonda BeLue

1.1   Global Health Collaboration

In the era of Sustainable Development Goals, multinational non-governmental organizations (NGOs), grand challenges, and record numbers of students seeking educational opportunities abroad, university global health partnerships are quickly becoming a mainstay (Merson 2014). These partnerships can bring together researchers, students, and community members in ways that address education, research, and community health needs. There are compelling advantages to having institutional partnerships so that individuals can collaborate to have a sustainable impact compared to working individually within institutions (Dockrell 2010). A collective base of expertise may also leverage scarce resources and help to develop creative solutions to intractable issues (Binagwaho et al. 2013). Frequently though, universities working together on these issues can reinforce existing disparities and unequal relationships that prioritize the flow of information, bodies, and agendas from higher to lower resourced parts of the globe (Crane 2010; Sewankambo et al. 2015; Syed et al. 2013).

We take as a starting point that partnerships, if built, maintained, and managed in an equitable fashion have the potential to generate a lasting positive impact on global health (Chu et al. 2014; Morse 2014; Pratt and Hyder 2016, 2017). The concept of reverse and global innovation flow is central to this equity, and prioritizes the knowledge and expertise from what is frequently referred to as the Global South (Syed et al. 2013; Crisp 2014). Reverse and global innovation flows create possibilities for relevant community-based research, open access dialogue, and

M. S. Winchester (✉) · C. Knapp
Health Policy and Administration, Pennsylvania State University, University Park, PA, USA
e-mail: winchester@psu.edu

R. BeLue
Health Management and Policy, St. Louis University, St. Louis, MO, USA

© The Author(s) 2018
M. S. Winchester et al. (eds.), *Global Health Collaboration*, SpringerBriefs in Public Health, https://doi.org/10.1007/978-3-319-77685-9_1

reciprocity and respect (Binagwaho et al. 2013; Crisp 2014; Snowdon et al. 2015). At a fundamental level, this is a challenge to the traditional dynamics of North-South models of collaboration. The global flow of ideas in the realm of health is by no means new, though typically only tacitly acknowledged when flowing in "reverse."

Given the ever-present community-academic and North-South imbalances, the Pan Institution Network for Global Health (PINGH)[1] employs a participatory governance and research approach to bring a balance of power by featuring local stakeholders as content and context experts. First, PINGH has a rotating governance structure. Each university partner has a champion who represents his/her institution for all PINGH activities. Second, leadership rotates on a three-year cycle. Each institution takes turns leading PINGH initiatives as well as hosting the annual PINGH collaborative meeting, in order to offer an opportunity for all PINGH members to experience and gain insight on the institutional and local cultures of each PINGH member and to defray costs of hosting the meeting for any one institution. These activities also insure participation and contribution from all PINGH members in the global North and South.

To promote inclusivity, we invite community stakeholders to our annual meetings to ensure that PINGH objectives are relevant to the local communities in which PINGH institutional members serve. Local NGOs, government policy makers, and other local stakeholders have attended PINGH meetings to help our partners reflect and strategize on how global health research and capacity building can be translated to local policy and practice. Our approach to community stakeholder involvement is discussed in further detail in this chapter.

1.2   History of PINGH

The Pan Institution Network for Global Health (PINGH) is the result of a targeted interest in using university partnerships to address global health needs (Winchester et al. 2016). In 2014, Pennsylvania State University hosted a meeting to discuss potential mechanisms and collaborations among more than a dozen global universities. After the meeting, faculty members across the universities established basic guidelines for working together, including a steering committee of 'champions' from each institution and two thematic priorities within the broader field of global health (detailed below). Following a consolidation of interest, the core membership of PINGH included six universities: Albert Ludwigs University of Freiburg (Germany), Savitribai Phule Pune University (India), The University of the West Indies (Barbados, Jamaica, and Trinidad and Tobago), University of Cape Town (South Africa), University of Limpopo (South Africa), and Pennsylvania State University. More recently, Mountcrest University (Ghana) has also joined the group.

Central to PINGH's vision are three pillars of collaboration: (1) research, (2) education, and (3) capacity building. Each of these pillars is dependent on the others

---

[1] Formerly the Pan University Network for Global Health (PUNGH).

and none represents the sole reason for the network. PINGH is still relatively young, but has a growing portfolio of activities within each area.

To encourage collaboration, PINGH leadership initiated several activities, including pilot projects. The pilot projects were intended to serve a dual purpose: First to encourage collaboration between PINGH members. Pilot project funding guidelines required that at least two PINGH members were included and at least one global South institution was included on every funded project. Secondly, pilot projects were selected to advance PINGH pillars. During the first two years after the network's founding, through funding from Pennsylvania State University, PINGH was able to offer two rounds of seed grants, totaling $100,000 USD. We funded 11 projects, described below. Many of these projects are also further detailed in subsequent chapters, including successes, challenges, and lessons learned.

Several grants were awarded in early 2014: three capacity building meetings, two secondary data analyses, and two primary research studies. One project organized a conference to establish a multidiscplinary network of emerging scholars on migration, urbanization and health in Southern Africa and included partners from Pennsylvania State University, University of Cape Town, and University of Witwatersrand. The group hosted a workshop in July 2015 that included three keynote presentations and ten presentations from early career researchers across Southern Africa. Pre- and post-workshop, emerging researchers were paired up with established scholars to exchange comments on drafts of papers, feedback on presentations, and even grant and publication opportunities. Another meeting was organized in Jamaica in April 2015 to facilitate writing and partnerships between investigators at Pennsylvania State University, the University of the West Indies, and University of Cape Town, and focused on the intersection of HIV and chronic diseases. The group completed a systematic review and have remained partners, submitting multiple grants together, and eventually combined with another project focused on improving systems for chronic care. The group studying the intersection of chronic and infectious diseases in health systems included partners from Pennsylvania State University, University of Limpopo, and University of Cape Town. They collected primary data, developed an optimization model for care, completed the training of two graduate students in public health, and have published one paper to date (Oni et al. 2014). Using existing data sets, another project examined the relationship between body mass index and mortality, with investigators from Pennsylvania State University, Savitribai Phule Pune University, Hebei Union University, and Kailuan Hospital. This project resulted in two peer-reviewed publications, but the investigators decided not to pursue an ongoing partnership (Cheng et al. 2016a, b). The other project using secondary data identified priority areas for mother and child interventions in Cape Town, with partners from Pennsylvania State University, University of Cape Town, University of Freiburg, and Savitribai Phule Pune University. As a result, the investigators have had ongoing partnerships with multiple grants submitted and one published paper to date (Mumm et al. 2017). One final project set out to develop new partnerships between Pennsylvania State University, Savitribai Phule Pune University, and the University of Cape Town to study vitamin D deficiency and pregnancy. This grant led to multiple meetings, but the group ultimately was unable to proceed with data collection for a variety of reasons.

In January 2016, a second round of five grants was funded. This round focused on scaling up existing research collaborations and building capacity among junior network members. These projects all required some sort of matching funds or resources in kind from partner institutions. The team that investigated the intersection of HIV and chronic diseases was funded a second time to study systems for strengthening chronic care in South Africa and the Caribbean, with partners from Pennsylvania State University, the University of the West Indies, University of Cape Town, and University of Limpopo. As a direct result of this project, two additional master of public health students were trained and several article manuscripts are in process. The group has identified external funding and will use the data collected as a pilot for this larger project to improve healthcare for multiple morbidities. Another research project with researchers at Pennsylvania State University and Savitribai Phule Pune University has been studying the healthcare access of informal workers in India and the United States. This group has collected data in New York, a student analyzed the data for a master's thesis in Health Policy and Administration, and the group is in the process of working with community partners to determine next steps. The 'Secret History' methodology is a South African-developed training for empathic healthcare; a group from University of Cape Town, University of Freiburg, and Pennsylvania State University was funded to bring this training to healthcare workers in Germany. The group conducted two sets of trainings, and then disseminated the information and additional training among PINGH members at one of the annual network meetings. Three papers from the trainings are in process, to detail the adaptation of the method across settings. Another group hosted a workshop on urbanization and health for young scholars and graduate students in Pune, India in early 2017. Attended by more than two dozen faculty, the workshop facilitated proposal writing and other urban health activities at Savitribai Phule Pune University. Finally, a small grant was given to faculty from Pennsylvania State University and Savitribai Phule Pune University to explore the development of online modules in public health and health systems. The group faced significant logistical difficulties in developing a formal course, but ended up collaborating in different ways, including the hosting of international public health students in India and reciprocal review of materials.

Some of these projects have blossomed into further ongoing partnerships and activities. PINGH members meet in person annually, in addition to regular electronic and video communication for projects and between champions. PINGH also encourages bilateral and smaller group collaborations. Global North-South bilateral relationships and projects are especially encouraged. Each of the member institutions has branched out to develop these relationships outside the network.

PINGH facilitates the development of global health infrastructure within each member institution. PINGH members are encouraged to strengthen global health activities within their own institutions and then share these strategies and activities with other PINGH members at annual meetings. Global health seminar series, global health policy workshops, and events offered at individual PINGH institutions are advertised through the PINGH newsletter and emails so that partner institutions may replicate in their own institutions. Bilateral relationships have included research projects, education and training initiatives, and student development such as participation as a reviewer, examiner or committee member on graduate student thesis and dissertation committees.

1.3   Priority Areas

Within the ever-expanding field of global health, PINGH has selected two specific priority areas: multiple morbidities and urban health. Both of these areas are in line with the shifting global burden of disease and growing population (Winchester et al. 2016). In today's globalized world, many low- and middle-income countries are undergoing rapid changes that are conducive to both ongoing infectious disease burdens and growing rates of noncommunicable diseases (Murray and Lopez 2013). In particular, rapid urbanization, mechanization of the rural economy, and the increasing activities of transnational food, drink, and tobacco corporations are all associated with behavioral changes that increase the risk of noncommunicable diseases. As a result, population health profiles and patterns are rapidly changing with an increase in cardiovascular and metabolic disorders. Population estimates suggest that by 2045 there will be over six billion urban residents, out of a global population of nine billion. The global, regional, and local variation in the trends we see today relating to shifting demographics and spatial inequalities ensure that the majority of population growth will occur in developing countries, with relative growth being highest across Africa. While megacities (the very largest global metropolises) are often highlighted, urban growth has occurred across the entire settlement system, reinforcing existing health challenges as well as generating new ones (Montgomery 2008). Processes of urbanization provide the dynamic backdrop to how we conceptualize and define global health challenges.

1.4   Framework and Guiding Principles

Guiding all of PINGH's activities and selection of priorities has been a commitment to equity, both in collaboration and global health more broadly. These two aims are deeply entwined and guide our governance practices within the network. We outline our logic model elsewhere (Winchester et al. 2016), but note that it is built on two assumptions: (1) that partnerships and the reciprocal flow of innovation is necessary to address global health and health care challenges, and (2) collaboration requires engaged network members, collective decision making and open communication. Building on Pratt and Hyder's (2017) framework for governance of global health consortia, we aim for a deliberate and inclusive process among our partners. They emphasize the two aspects of shared sovereignty and shared resources, as the foundation of equitable partnerships. While PINGH's founding was initiated by one US-based university, we have actively sought to include representatives from each institution in a single governing board. Partners have nominated a 'champion' for their university, and this person is part of the network's governing board. Champions are chosen for their standing within the institution, ability to connect interested faculty, and to potentially garner resources. The board has one director, currently at Pennsylvania State University, where there is also a full time faculty coordinator for managing network activities. In order to maintain equity among members, we are moving to a rotating model, which will allow each institution to take up to a three-year term 'hosting' the network, directorship, and coordination. Not all partners have access to similar levels of resources at their institutions, and may opt for a shorter term.

In keeping with our goal to conduct research that can be readily translated to policy, advocacy, and practice, we include community partners, practitioners, and government representatives at all of our meetings. We follow the Health in All Policies (HiAP) approach (WHO 2014), which posits that policies made in all sectors can significantly affect population health and health equity. In a global and interconnected society, health is influenced by demographic, environmental, and social forces. In the spirit of the HiAP framework, at our annual meetings and all PINGH sponsored events, we include not only local stakeholders that represent health care organizations, but stakeholders who represent social, environmental, transportation, and economic sectors that affect health through social processes. Inviting a diverse group of local stakeholders also offers an opportunity for PINGH colleagues from other countries to more deeply understand the sociopolitical dynamics of their collaborators' countries which facilitates improved and more informed research collaborations.

1.5 Outline of Chapters and Volume

Each chapter in this edited volume showcases one project or aspect of a project completed by PINGH members. While there are many intersections and overlaps among the projects and authors, we have divided up the sections to focus on lessons learned through specific activities. We are the first to admit that PINGH is still a young network and we are still learning. The chapters each focus on lessons learned through trial and error. While some groups have been able to establish best practices, others share the challenges and pitfalls that can happen when working across contexts and how to avoid replicating our mistakes.

This book consists of two sections that provide case studies, evidence, and experiences related to essential elements of the PINGH model of cross-national partnerships including education, capacity building, and research. The first section focuses specifically on the PINGH education and capacity building pillars. Chapters focus on strategies and lessons learned related to global health education for diverse students, the process of building collaborative research capacity to effectively study the effects of urbanization, and the cultural and contextual adaptation of women's health care training protocols from the global south to the global north. The final section of the Education and Collaboration section discusses strategies to sustain and finance global health collaboration.

The second section entitled Research Lessons consists of case studies and lessons learned from cross-national research initiatives that were initiated through PINGH pilot project funding. These chapters present work directly related to our research foci: multiple morbidity and urbanization. All case studies approach research from a cross-national perspective. The first chapter of this section, Chap. 5, explores the concept of patient workload in relation to managing multiple chronic illnesses, specifically HIV and Diabetes. Chapters 6 and 7 explore urbanization from two points of view. First is a cross-national study on challenges and needs of informal wastepickers in urban context. Second, is the application of a maternal-child health research framework for identifying maternal child health resources in urban areas, and how this framework can be applied to broad urban settings. The concluding chapter discusses ways forward and long-term needs to advance global health research and collaborations. Lastly, this edited volume ends with a personal reflection from a long time global health scholar and the founder of the PINGH network.

References

Binagwaho A, Nutt CT, Mutabazi V, Karema C et al (2013) Shared learning in an interconnected world: innovations to advance global health equity. Global Health 9(1):37. doi. org/10.1186/1744-8603-9-37

Cheng FW, Gao X, Mitchell DC et al (2016a) Body mass index and all-cause mortality among older adults. Obesity 24(10):2232–2239. https://doi.org/10.1002/oby.21612

Cheng FW, Gao X, Mitchell DC et al (2016b) Metabolic health status and the obesity paradox in older adults. J Nutr Gerontol Geriatr 35(3):161–176. https://doi.org/10.1080/21551197.2016.1199004

Chu KM, Jayaraman S, Kyamanywa P et al (2014) Building research capacity in Africa: equity and global health collaborations. PLOS Med 11(3):e1001612. doi.org/10.1371/journal.pmed.1001612

Crane JT (2010) Unequal 'partners.' AIDS, academia, and the rise of global health. Behemoth–a Journal on Civilisation 3(3):78–97. doi.org/10.6094/behemoth.2010.3.3.685

Crisp N (2014) Mutual learning and reverse innovation–where next? Global Health 10(1):14. doi. org/10.1186/1744-8603-10-14

Dockrell HM (2010) Presidential address: the role of research networks in tackling major challenges in international health. Int Health 2(3):181–185. doi.org/10.1016/j.inhe.2010.07.004

Merson MH (2014) University engagement in global health. N Engl J Med 370(18):1676. https://doi.org/10.1056/NEJMp1401124

Montgomery MR (2008) The urban transformation of the developing world. Science 319(5864):761–764. https://doi.org/10.1126/science.1153012

Morse M (2014) Responsible global health engagement: A road map to equity for academic partnerships. J Grad Med Educ 6(2):347–348. doi.org/10.4300/JGME-D-14-00165.1

Mumm R, Diaz-Monsalve S, Hänselmann E et al (2017) Exploring urban health in Cape Town, South Africa: an interdisciplinary analysis of secondary data. Pathog Glob Health 111(1):7–22. dx.doi.org/10.1080/20477724.2016.1275463

Murray CJ, Lopez AD (2013) Measuring the global burden of disease. N Engl J Med, 369(5):448–457

Oni T, McGrath N, BeLue R et al (2014) Chronic diseases and multi-morbidity–a conceptual modification to the WHO ICCC model for countries in health transition. BMC Public Health 14(1):575. doi.org/10.1186/1471-2458-14-575

Pratt B, Hyder AA (2016) Governance of transnational global health research consortia and health equity. Am J Bioeth 16(10):29–45. dx.doi.org/10.1080/15265161.2016.1214304

Pratt B, Hyder AA (2017) Governance of global health research consortia: sharing sovereignty and resources within future health systems. Soc Sci Med 174:113–121. doi.org/10.1016/j. socscimed.2016.11.039

Sewankambo N, Tumwine JK, Tomson G et al (2015) Enabling dynamic partnerships through joint degrees between low- and high-income countries for capacity development in global health research: experience from the Karolinska Institutet/Makerere University partnership. PLOS Med 12(2):e1001784. doi.org/10.1371/journal.pmed.1001784

Snowdon AW, Bassi H, Scarffe AD et al (2015) Reverse innovation: an opportunity for strengthening health systems. Global Health 11(1):2. doi.org/10.1186/s12992-015-0088-x

Syed SB, Dadwal V, Martin G (2013) Reverse innovation in global health systems: towards global innovation flow. Global Health 9(1):36. doi.org/10.1186/1744-8603-9-36

Winchester MS, BeLue R, Oni T et al (2016) The Pan-University Network for Global Health: framework for collaboration and review of global health needs. Global Health 12(1):13. doi. org/10.1186/s12992-016-0151-2

World Health Organization (2014) Health in all policies: Helsinki statement. Framework for country action. http://apps.who.int/iris/bitstream/10665/112636/1/9789241506908_eng.pdf. Accessed 30 Oct 2017

Chapter 2
Connecting the Dots: Cultivating a Sustainable Interdisciplinary Discourse Around Migration, Urbanisation, and Health in Southern Africa

Jo Hunter-Adams, Tackson Makandwa, Stephen A. Matthews, Henrietta Nyamnjoh, Tolu Oni, and Jo Vearey

2.1 Introduction

Migration and urbanisation attract much interest globally, reflecting growing concerns associated with the management of urban growth (UN-Habitat 2016) and, increasingly, around the ways in which these social and demographic processes are associated with health and wellbeing (Galea and Vladhov 2005; Grant et al. 2017; Nauman et al. 2016). Recognising that there are complex – but poorly understood – linkages between migration, urbanisation and health globally, the key elements of an emerging research agenda have recently begun to be mapped out (Grant et al. 2017; IOM 2016; Hanefeld et al. 2017). However – with few notable exceptions (Oni et al. 2016) – these agendas tend to focus on ways in which migration *or* urbanisation is associated with health, and are insufficiently Africa-oriented. In an attempt to contribute to addressing this gap, we use this chapter to reflect on our experiences in supporting early-career scholars to further the research agenda associated with migration, urbanisation and health in Southern African Development Community (SADC).

All authors contributed equally

J. Hunter-Adams (✉) · T. Oni
School of Public Health and Family Medicine, University of Cape Town,
Cape Town, Republic of South Africa

T. Makandwa · J. Vearey
African Centre for Migration & Society, University of the Witwatersrand,
Johannesburg, Republic of South Africa

S. A. Matthews
Population Research Institute, Pennsylvania State University, State College, PA, USA

H. Nyamnjoh
African Centre for Cities, University of Cape Town, Cape Town, Republic of South Africa

© The Author(s) 2018
M. S. Winchester et al. (eds.), *Global Health Collaboration*, SpringerBriefs
in Public Health, https://doi.org/10.1007/978-3-319-77685-9_2

The SADC population is expected to double from 250 million to approximately 500 million people by 2040 (IOM 2010) and, by 2035, over 50% of the population is anticipated to reside in cities (UN 2014). The region is associated with high levels of historical and contemporary population movements including internal migration – dominated by movement between rural and urban spaces, and increasingly by inter- and intra-urban movements; cross-border migration from neighbouring countries; and long distance moves within and between continents (Walls et al. 2016). Additionally, the region is associated with a high prevalence of communicable diseases – notably HIV, tuberculosis (TB) and malaria, – and an increasing burden of non-communicable diseases (NCDs), mental ill-health, and injury (McMichael 2000; Vearey 2014). The public health systems of member states are struggling, creating additional tensions when exploring the intersections between migration, urbanisation and health (Vearey 2014), and researchers and policy makers increasingly recognise the need to better understand these complex linkages (Vearey 2014; Walls et al. 2016). This is particularly relevant when working to improve intersectoral responses to ensure that 'no-one is left behind' when working to achieve good health for all (United Nations 2016). In this chapter, we focus on the case of South Africa (SA) for several reasons: it is the most urbanised country in SADC; it receives the largest number of cross-border migrants within the region; it is home to a large internal migrant population that far outnumbers cross-border migrants; and, it bears a high communicable – and an increasing NCD – burden (Vearey 2014). However, regional research focuses on SA, producing a lopsided view of the region – highlighting the need for renewed research focus in other SADC member states.

Migration is a central determinant of health We consider migration a central determinant of health, and recognise the complex bidirectional relationship at play: migration can affect health, and health status can affect decisions to move (Castañeda et al. 2015; Davies et al. 2009; Vearey 2014). Given this, and the knowledge that healthy migration is good for development (Vearey 2014; IOM 2010), it is surprising that existing health responses at regional and country levels do not adequately engage with and respond to migration, mobility and urbanisation (Walls et al. 2016; Vearey et al. 2017). Despite being positively selected and often being in better health than the host population at their time of arrival in the city, some migrant groups – including both internal and cross-border migrants – experience an 'urban health penalty' due to their exposure to unhealthy physical and social conditions, and uneven landscapes of risk in the urban context (Carballo and Nerukar 2001; Freudenberg et al. 2005). These inequitable outcomes in poor health manifest in both urban and rural areas, where the burden of sick migrants returning home to receive care is borne by the sending households and (often rural) healthcare systems (Carballo and Nerukar 2001).

Demographic Shifts Migration is generally a selective process, with migrants clustering in specific economic and reproductive age groups, which influences fertility rates in receiving areas (StatsSA 2011). Both internal and cross border migrants affect the demographic composition of destination countries, provinces and municipalities, such that the compositional heterogeneity of the population changes– by age, gender, ethnicity and socioeconomic position – exacerbating the appropriateness of the services provided (Morrison 1979; Gelatt et al. 2014). Changing age and gender compositions are interconnected with emerging challenges related to new health and disease (mortality and morbidity) profiles, social gradients of health, and the provisioning of equitable levels of service for preventive and reproductive health (Marmot 2004).

A range of socio-political, economic and demographic factors have led to the movement of people within the SADC region, and the associated growth observed in urban areas (Vearey 2013). This is associated with a growing population of the 'urban poor' and vulnerable subgroups, many of whom are recent migrants to the city and occupy the peripheries, with marginal access to health and social welfare (Vearey 2010, 2013). Key concerns relate to a lack of focus on the social determinants of urban health as well as the lack of effective management of chronic conditions – including communicable diseases – for those who move (Sargent and Larchanche 2011). This has negative public health implications, affecting the morbidity and mortality of a highly mobile population in both urban and rural areas (Vearey 2014), and on those who do not move (Gushulak and MacPherson 2006). These negative implications extend beyond the individual, and include the healthcare systems and family structures that are forced to manage the costs associated with the current limited responses to migration and health in the region (IOM 2010).

South Africa South African cities present unique spaces within which to explore the complex and multidirectional ways in which migration, urbanisation and health are connected, as the country is witnessing multiple simultaneous and interconnected transitions (health, demographic, social, economic and political). Before democracy, the apartheid government promoted racial/spatial segregation, restricted and controlled movement of people internally and across borders– resulting in distorted urbanisation, and today's pattern of intra-urban disparities and inequities in health. The transition to democracy in SA provided a new context for the process of urbanisation as free movement for the local population was guaranteed and cross-border migration increased due to the search for improved livelihood opportunities and political unrest in neighbouring countries (Landau and Segatti 2011). Today, cross border migrants arriving in South Africa are diverse and include highly-skilled and low-skilled immigrants, refugees, asylum seekers, and other documented and undocumented migrants (Landau and Segatti 2011).

2.2   A Workshop for Interdisciplinary Discussion of Migration, Urbanisation, and Health

The dynamics of urbanisation and migration, and their implications for health in the SADC region, led researchers from the University of the Witwatersrand (WITS), the University of Cape Town, and Pennsylvania State University to convene a 3-day meeting in July 2015. The workshop brought together senior and early-career scholars working on urban and/or migration and health across the social and health sciences, to discuss ways of engaging with migration and health in the context of urbanisation in SADC. Once abstracts were accepted for presentation, presenting early-career scholars were matched with the four workshop organisers who provided feedback on papers before the workshop. The workshop privileged emerging scholars; there were ten in total: five doctoral students whose presentations focused on their dissertations; three post-doctoral researchers; and, two MA graduates—one working as a researcher and one in a non-governmental organisation.

The workshop aimed to understand the current social and political contexts shaping migrant health, migration trajectories and health histories; the lived experiences of urban (internal and cross-border) migrants and the ways in which these lived experiences can shape the research agenda with regard to health; and, how current policy and practice can contribute to migrant well-being or marginality. The workshop was guided by four overarching questions:

1. What are the current social and political contexts shaping the health of migrants[1] in SADC?
2. What are the migration trajectories, health histories and lived experiences of urban migrants – with a focus of comparing long-term residents with new arrivals – within SADC?
3. How does current policy and practice contribute to migrant wellbeing or marginality in SADC?
4. How should what is known about the lived experiences of migrants contribute to the urban health research agenda, and how should insights emerging from this agenda inform the migration and health agenda?

These questions informed discussions around three key themes – access, lived experiences, and governance – that are described below.

Access Access refers to a range of positive determinants of health, including healthcare, social services or the realisation of food security. Presentations and discussions highlighted multiple forms of marginalisation in urban areas of SA, including of Zimbabwean, Cameroonian, Congolese (Democratic Republic of Congo – DRC) and internal migrants. Migrants are often marginalised and devalued, including when accessing healthcare; and – as a result – may turn to clinics and hospitals only as a last resort, especially female migrants during pregnancy and childbirth. Despite the availability of healthcare facilities they may be underutilised by some migrant groups due to previous negative experiences, or for fear of deportation associated with a lack of documentation required to be in the country legally. These fears are fanned by a lack of political voice, representation and legal protection among migrant population. The political contexts that migrants operate in are inhospitable and hinder maintenance of optimal health and health seeking behaviours. Significantly, a number of healthcare barriers impeding migrant access to healthcare were identified. These include the nature of their employment, language, power relations, and discrimination on the basis of nationality or place of origin.

---

[1] Migrants refers to both cross-border and internal migrant groups.

Lived Experiences The challenges of realising good health in an urban context affect both internal and cross-border migrants. These challenges include poor mental health; mediated by education level, marital status and socio-economic situation, as well as country or province of origin. The urban environment contributes to growing inequity in wellbeing; in the case of peripheral urban spaces, economic, social and physical changes over the past few decades have reinforced marginalisation. Pathways that affect the health of migrants living on the periphery relate to unemployment and crime; inadequate shelter, infrastructure and services; a complex food environment in which it is difficult to achieve food security; a built environment that is not conducive to safe physical activity; and high levels of depression and stress – linked to, poverty, crime and fear of crime and deportation. Improving the understanding of lived experiences requires engagement with differing understandings of health and ill health, and alternative health and help-seeking strategies, such as churches and community support – including from others from their country of origin, and from those back home.

Role of Governance and Policy A key focus of many researchers at the symposium was on how cross-border migrants navigate and negotiate healthcare in public facilities and in turn how migrants are perceived as a public health threat or a liability by the state, by healthcare professionals and by local citizens. Securitisation with regard to migration is not limited to border control but extends to the (increasing) securitisation of healthcare and communicable diseases surveillance in SA. This is despite the fact that, often, rather than bringing communicable diseases, it is the marginalisation that cross-border and internal migrants face in SA cities that can put them at risk of contracting communicable diseases *after* arriving in the city. Migrants' well-being in host societies is partly informed by the extent to which they can access healthcare and other social services, safe housing, and secure livelihoods.

One important dimension of speaking to policy involved the explicit definition and consideration of contested terms. For example, it was vital to engage in a discussion of what is meant by human mobility. In SADC, this was determined to encompasses travel that is circular and involves cycles of return that can be rapid (daily, weekly, monthly), as well as more permanent movement (annual trips home, or even less frequently). Mobility in the region is still dominated by working-aged individuals and families, meaning that issues related to maternal and child health remain important focal areas for consideration. Furthermore, the legal experience of those who migrate relates to health. For example, the category of refugee has (unevenly) invoked legal protection, and also specific health responses on the part of the state.

2.3 Towards a Collective Agenda: Connecting the Dots

We wanted to tap into the research emerging from multiple disciplines in order to 'connect the dots': to identify the overlapping research and policy priorities surrounding migration, urbanisation and health more effectively. During the

Table 2.1 Towards an emerging research agenda on migration, urbanisation and health in SADC

Key issue	Some key considerations
We need to establish common definitions of key concepts.	Urban/rural; mobility; migration; health; medical; traditional; urban advantage; urban health penalty; resilience
We need to better understand the complex contexts in which we work.	Legal frameworks; epidemiological profiles; working/living/travelling environments; social determinants of (urban) health framework; role of social networks; social capital
We need to acknowledge and engage with the heterogeneity of movement and mobility.	Daily; weekly; monthly; circular, categories of migrant; age; sex; moving alone; moving with family; forced movements; livelihood seeking movement
We need to better understand the lived experiences of people who move and enter the urban space.	Heterogeneity; migration trajectories; urbanisation experiences; embodied experiences
We need to enact a holistic view of health and wellbeing, and move away from the prevailing focus on access to biomedical services.	Plural health systems; understandings of health and wellbeing; idioms of distress; somatisation
We need to develop more effective ways for translating research into policy.	Engagement with the state – empirically and in practice; exploring ways of generating and communicating research; involved research approaches
We need to develop improved, pragmatic and interdisciplinary methodologies to address the concerns identified above.	Engaging with complexity; quantitative; qualitative; involved research practice; working with communities to co-develop and co-produce research; visual; medical; multiple places; comparative; place-based approaches; research along migration trajectories

workshop organizing process, we identified the importance of cultivating a network through which to communicate and continue to grapple with the identified policy and research themes. The *Migration, Urbanisation and Health Network (HumNet)* aims to provide a virtual way of continuing the conversation started in the workshop, and for ongoing support to early career scholars. A key concern identified in the workshop revolved around the idea of how to use our research to inform policy and practice. For example, we discussed concepts and definitions as they applied to the lived experiences of migrants in the SADC region. A central theme that emerged was in foregrounding community-based research, and in unpacking the layers of connections between emerging researchers, more established researchers, policy makers, and civil society. Some of the key issues identified for an emerging research agenda on migration, urbanisation and health in SADC are presented in Table 2.1. The issues are identified are a guide only; it is essential that the key concerns are mapped for different contexts.

Scholars working on migration, urbanisation and health come from many different disciplinary traditions. It is vital that we find a common language to allow our research to be understood across disciplines. Meaningfully engaging across disciplines—as was the case in this workshop—requires methodological pragmatism and plain language. We discussed the use of methodologies that unpack our disciplinary jargon and allow us to engage in the complexity of migration, experimenting with terms and language that best captured the contexts and audiences in our region. For example, the term migration itself comes with particular preconceptions of human movement in a particular region. For us, it was valuable to consider the role of circular migration in mediating (poor) health outcomes in both sending and receiving communities.

Considering various ways of approaching migration in the region represented a first effort to engage and connect different people who can contribute to research, policy, and practice related to migration, urbanisation and health. At our meeting, the main focus was figuring out ways to speak that were less alienating to those engaged in practice, and those for whom urban or migrant health was a more peripheral part of their work. There needs to be multiple layers of engagement and multiple entry points into understanding linkages between migration, urbanisation and health in SADC—from research that serves to dispel myths, to that which builds much deeper knowledge in the region.

In addition to exploring ways to use language and approaches that not only speak across disciplines, we wished to understand ways to directly engage with those who are mobile, and who may experience health penalties as a result of their mobility or migration status. These methods should—we felt—be participatory, highly local, and support participatory action. Our focus on local, rather than reproducible, large scale, or transferable, kinds of knowledge, reflected a need to understand and foreground our local context. Place-based contextual knowledge allows for opportunities to connect and understand local policy and practice. Being connected to and engaging with the state is vital in our research, as the state is a key actor – both in defining who migrates, and in defining their experience of migration.

2.4 Cultivating a Sustainable Interdisciplinary Conversation

Migration, urbanisation and health are important contemporary social challenges and – as reflected in the diverse themes shared at the workshop – these challenges are dynamic. While a single disciplinary focus may be able to etch out small incremental gains in knowledge, there is a general recognition that collaboration across disciplines has the potential to be transformative, generate innovative ideas – and even solutions, and ultimately improve collective understanding of the most important real world problems (Ledford 2015). Interdisciplinary perspectives are especially relevant when examining the influence of global, national and local processes on individual outcomes, and in circumstances where the core policy and research questions require an analysis of complex patterns of interrelated social, behavioural, health, economic, and environmental phenomena – as in the general focus on the theme of migration, urbanisation and health.

Recognising the need for sustainable interdisciplinary research and facilitating it are, however, two different things. There are certainly risks to interdisciplinary collaboration, not least of which is the lack of incentives to engage in such collaboration (van Rijnsoever and Hessels 2011). But big questions require closer integration across disciplines on concepts, data, and methods – as well as multilevel and multi-sectoral frameworks of analysis. It is then necessary to discuss the benefits, risks and challenges for the current and next-generation of scholars and to identify mechanisms that can promote readiness for collaboration.

As implied above, big questions require big ideas or frameworks, and specifically frameworks that are seemingly holistic and flexible; frameworks are not static and should be utilised as a tool to assist in the development of relevant research agendas. Fortunately for urban health researchers, several inclusive frameworks already exist and it was evident at the workshop that all participants comfortably fit under the umbrella of the 'Social Determinants of Health' (SDH) or similarly multilevel and multisectoral frameworks.

If sustainable interdisciplinary research requires a common set of critical questions and an integrative framework, then the study of urbanisation, migration and health is ideal -providing opportunities to transcend disciplinary perspectives and silos (Syme 2008) and seeds have already been sown for promoting interdisciplinary research in undergraduate and postgraduate training programmes around questions of society and human health. However, there is always room for reframing and extending opportunities promoting interdisciplinary research and for hearing the perspective from early-career researchers in this field. It was with this in mind that our workshop helped foster interdisciplinary engagement—sharing ideas in an open forum and exploring collaboration—around urbanisation, migration and health.

While senior scholars collaborated to organize and frame the event, the workshop focused on presentations by two distinct groups of participants: early-career scholars presenting their *own* work, and inputs from invited speakers whose work transcended the academic and policy divide. The involvement of participants from outside academia can contextualise and provide alternative views on a 'real-world' problem. This workshop structure reflected ideas reported in the literature where promoting the opportunity for interdisciplinary, multisector *encounters* and supporting open communication in both formal and informal (and unstructured) settings are an effective means to facilitate the development of future interdisciplinary researchers (Bridle et al. 2013).

Bridle et al. (2013) distinguish between "*cultivation*" and "*development*" encounters. Cultivation encounters are designed to expose researchers who are not yet involved in interdisciplinary projects to other disciplines, perspectives, concepts, ideas, measures, language, approaches, and tools as well as to help participants to understand what those disciplines have to offer and to explore potential areas of collaboration. Follow-up encounters are more likely framed as development encounters, where the premise is that people are brought together to generate new ideas or initiate concrete collaborative outputs—joint research papers and or funding proposals.

Our workshop touched on both the cultivation and development aspects of promoting collaboration across fields. While individual early career scholars came to the table with their own work and perspectives, the diversity of topics, research methods, and levels of integration with policy and legal actors across the sessions was impressive (see Table 2.1). This diverse coverage reflects the idea of cultivation; when we reflected as a group on the issues identified during the workshop, it was evident that there was both common ground and areas of intersection but also much to be learned from each other. A short term outcome of the meeting linked to the opportunities for the early-career scholars to improve and refine their communication skills when presenting their own work to a diverse audience, as well as for some the opportunity to lead and facilitate group discussions.

The challenge is to move to the next step, explicitly focusing on further encounters to develop and sustain capacity within SADC to influence research and public policy. While interdisciplinary research can have considerable benefits it can also incur substantial costs, owing to the need to invest significant time in building truly collaborative relationships, developing shared language and honing a common perspective from disparate viewpoints (Bromham et al. 2016).

We have made concerted efforts to promote the transfer of knowledge and information from the established to the early-career scholars that attended the workshop, and these have focused on topics related to research practice within academia, the interface with public policy, and community engagement – as well other components of professional development such as sharing calls for papers, conference announcements, and strategies for publishing. The exchange of ideas and practice vis-à-vis professional development, while it may be asymmetrical between established and early-career scholars, should not be one way. Emerging areas of research and new ideas (e.g., lived experiences), new measurement and data needs (e.g., capturing the heterogeneity of mobility), contexts (e.g., legal environments) and new research methods (e.g., visual) and the integration of mixed methods (Hesse-Biber and Johnson 2015) can be areas where innovation is spurred on by the next generation of scholars. Among the many strategies to be simultaneously explored, we would prioritise training and instruction – specifically the provisioning of opportunities related to early-career development such as post-doctoral fellowships, exchange visits between departments, institutes and universities during both graduate and postgraduate studies, as well as exploring the placement of scholars within government and non-government agencies. We see opportunities for mentoring and exchange between all levels of the academy and with non-academic partners. Technology – emails, listserves, blogs[2] and social media[3,4] – offers a vehicle for new ways of sharing and collaborating but face-to-face meetings can build better and more sustainable teams. Collectively, we continue to promote cultivating links and development opportunities as the *Migration, Urbanisation and Health Network (HumNet)* but we have a long way to go.

Challenges
- Scholars working on migration, urbanisation and health come from many different disciplinary traditions. It is vital that we find a common language to allow our research to be understood across disciplines.

---

[2] http://migrationurbanisationhealth.tumblr.com/.

[3] https://goo.gl/bSD8ti.

[4] https://twitter.com/HumNet2015.

- There needs to be multiple layers of engagement and multiple entry points into understanding linkages between migration, urbanisation and health in SADC—from research that serves to dispel myths, to that which builds much deeper knowledge in the region.
- We need to develop more effective ways for translating research into policy.

Lessons Learned

- Our focus on local, rather than reproducible, large scale, or transferable, kinds of knowledge, reflected a need to understand and foreground our local context. Place-based contextual knowledge allows for opportunities to connect and understand local policy and practice.
- Our workshop structure that prioritized emerging researchers and connections with policy makers facilitated dialogue between groups and allowed for both formal and informal conversations about creating bridges between the two.
- Technology offers a vehicle for new ways of sharing and collaborating but face-to-face meetings can build better and more sustainable teams.

Acknowledgements We thank all early career scholars who – in addition to the authors – participated in the workshop: Chukwuedozie Ajaero, Bailey Balekang, Lynlee Howard-Payne, Dostin Lakika, Erica Penfold, Stephen Pentz, Eva Roka and Theresa Sommers. Cath Burns, Sarah Charlton, Bronwyn Harris, Zaheera Jinnah, Lorena Nunez, and Warren Smit are thanked for their generous time and support to the workshop through acting as keynote speakers and respondents. Lenore Longwe is thanked for logistical support.

References

Bridle H, Vrieling A, Cardillo M et al (2013) Preparing for an interdisciplinary future: a perspective from early-career researchers. Futures 53:22–32. https://doi.org/10.1016/j.futures.2013.09.003

Bromham L, Dinnage R, Hua X (2016) Interdisciplinary research has consistently lower funding success. Nature 534:684–687. https://doi.org/10.1038/nature18315

Carballo M, Nerukar A (2001) Migration, refugees, and health risks. Emerg Infect Dis 7:556–560. https://doi.org/10.3201/eid0707.017733

Castañeda H, Holmes SM, Madrigal DS et al (2015) Immigration as a social determinant of health. Annu Rev Public Health 36:375–392. https://doi.org/10.1146/annurev-publhealth-032013-182419

Davies AA, Basten A, Frattini C (2009) Migration: a social determinant of the health of migrants. Eur Secur 16(1):10–12

Freudenberg N, Galea S, Vlahov D (2005) Beyond urban penalty and urban sprawl: back to living conditions as the focus of urban health. J Community Health 30(1):1–11. https://doi.org/10.1007/s10900-004-6091-4

Galea S, Vladhov D (2005) Urban health: evidence, challenges and directions. Annu Rev Public Health 26:341–365. https://doi.org/10.1146/annurev.publhealth.26.021304.144708

Gelatt J, Adams G, Monson W (2014) Immigration and the changing landscape for local service delivery: demographic shifts in cities and neighborhoods. The Urban Institute https://wwwurbanorg/sites/default/files/publication/22401/413062-Immigration-and-the-Changing-Landscape-for-Local-Service-DeliveryPDF. Accessed 2 Nov 2017

Grant M, Brown C, Caiaffa WT et al (2017) Cities and health: an evolving global conversation. Cities Health 1:1–9. https://doi.org/10.1080/23748834.2017.1316025

Gushulak BD, MacPherson DW (2006) The basic principles of migration health: population mobility and gaps in disease prevalence. Emerg Themes Epidemiol 3(1):3. https://doi.org/10.1186/1742-7622-3-3

Hanefeld J, Vearey J, Lunt N et al (2017) A global research agenda on migration, mobility, and health. Lancet 389:2358–2359. https://doi.org/10.1016/S0140-6736(17)31588-X

Hesse-Biber S, Johnson RB (eds) (2015) The Oxford handbook of multimethod and mixed methods research inquiry. Oxford University Press, Oxford, UK

IOM (2010) Migration and health in South Africa: a review of the current situation and recommendations for achieving the World Health Assembly Resolution on the health of migrants. IOM Regional Office for Southern Africa, Johannesburg

International Organization of Migration (2016) Concept note 2nd global consultation on migrant health: resetting the agenda. Colombo, International Organization of Migration

Landau L, Segatti A (2011) Contemporary migration to South Africa: a regional development issue. Africa development forum. World Bank, Washington, DC. http://documents.worldbank.org/curated/en/943521468101356700/Contemporary-migration-to-South-Africa-a-regional-development-issue. Accessed 25 Oct 2017

Ledford H (2015) How to solve the world's biggest problems. Nature 525:308–311. https://doi.org/10.1038/525308a

McMichael AJ (2000) The urban environment and health in a world of increasing globalization: issues for developing countries. Bull World Health Organ 78(9):1117–1126

Marmot M (2004) The status syndrome: how social standing affects our health and longevity. Henry Holt, New York

Morrison PA (1979) The future demographic context of the health care delivery system. RAND Corporation, Santa Monica

Nauman E, VanLandingham M, Anglewicz P (2016) Migration, urbanization and health. In: White MJ (ed) International handbook of migration and population distribution, International handbooks of population, vol 6. Springer, Dordrecht, pp 451–463. https://doi.org/10.1007/978-94-017-7282-2_20

Oni T, Smit W, Matzopoulos R et al (2016) Urban health research in Africa: themes and priority research questions. J Urban Health 93(4):722–730. https://doi.org/10.1007/s11524-016-0050-0

Sargent C, Larchanche S (2011) Transnational migration and global health: the production and management of risk, illness and access to care. Annu Rev Anthropol 40:345–361. https://doi.org/10.1146/annurev-anthro-081309-145811

StatsSA (2011) Census 2011 migration dynamics in South Africa. Statistics South Africa, Pretoria. http://www.statssa.gov.za/publications/Report-03-01-79/Report-03-01-792011.pdf. Accessed 25 Oct 2017. ISBN: 978-0-621-44166-6

Syme L (2008) The science of team science: assessing the value of transdisciplinary research. Am J Prev Med 35(2S):S94–S95. https://doi.org/10.1016/j.amepre.2008.05.017

United Nations, Department of Economic and Social Affairs, Population Division (2014) World urbanization prospects: the 2014 revision, highlights (ST/ESA/SER.A/352) United Nations, New York. http://esa.un.org/unpd/wup/Highlights/WUP2014-Highlights.pdf. Accessed 22 May 2017

United Nations, Department of Economic and Social Affairs (2016) Leaving no one behind: the imperative of inclusive development. Report on the world social situation 2016. (ST/ESA/362) United Nations, New York. http://www.un.org/esa/socdev/rwss/2016/full-report.pdf. Accessed 25 Oct 2017

UN-Habitat (2016) Urbanization and development: emerging futures. World cities report 2016 UN-Habitat, Nairobi. https://unhabitat.org/wp-content/uploads/2014/03/WCR-%20Full-Report-2016.pdf. Accessed 25 Oct 2017

Van Rijnsoever FJ, Hessles LK (2011) Factors associated with disciplinary and interdisciplinary research collaboration. Res Policy 40:463–472. https://doi.org/10.1016/j.respol.2010.11.001

Vearey J (2010) Hidden spaces and urban health: exploring the tactics of rural migrants navigating the city of gold. Urban Forum 21:37–53. https://doi.org/10.1007/s12132-010-9079-4

Vearey J (2013) Migration, urban health and inequality in Johannesburg. In: Bastia T (ed) Migration and inequality. Routledge, London, pp 121–144

Vearey J (2014) Healthy migration: a public health and development imperative for South(ern) Africa. S Afr Med J 104(10):663–664. https://doi.org/10.7196/SAMJ.8569

Vearey J, Modisenyane M, Hunter-Adams J (2017) Towards a migration-aware health system in South Africa: a strategic opportunity to address health inequity. In: Padarath A, Barron P (eds) South African health review. Health Systems Trust, Durban, pp 89–98. http://www.hst.org.za/publications/South%20African%20Health%20Reviews/HST%20SAHR%202017%20Web%20Version.pdf. Accessed 25 Oct 2017

Walls H, Vearey J, Modisenyane M et al (2016) Understanding healthcare and population mobility in southern Africa: the case of South Africa. S Afr Med J 106(1):14–15. https://doi.org/10.7196/SAMJ.2016.v106i1.10210

Chapter 3
Fostering Dialogues in Global Health Education: A Graduate and Undergraduate Approach

Kristin Sznajder, Dana Naughton, Anita Kar, Aarti Nagakar, Joyce Mashamba, Linda Shuro, Sebalda Leshabari, and Fatou Diop

3.1 Background

Worldwide, there are new public health threats due to urbanization, climate change, demographic shifts, globalization, and political climates. At the same time, the global public health workforce may be ill-equipped to manage these threats. The current global health academic landscape in high income countries (HICs), has seen expansive growth in developing undergraduate and graduate learning opportunities aimed to provide short-term immersion in low and middle income countries [(LMICs) Jogerst et al. 2015; Panosian and Coates 2006].

There are many well-documented benefits to global health educational partnerships between the global north and global south and university linkages are a major avenue for these collaborations. For universities or host institutions in the global

K. Sznajder (✉)
Public Health Sciences, The Pennsylvania State University, Hershey, PA, USA
e-mail: ksznajde@phs.psu.edu

D. Naughton
Department of Biobehavioral Health, The Pennsylvania State University,
University Park, PA, USA

A. Kar · A. Nagakar
Interdisciplinary School of Science, Savitribai Phule Pune University,
Pune, Maharashtra, India

J. Mashamba · L. Shuro
Health Promotion Unit, School of Public Health, University of Limpopo,
Polokwane, South Africa

S. Leshabari
Muhumbili University of Health and Allied Sciences, Dar es Salaam, Tanzania

F. Diop
Mbour Hospital, Mbour, Senegal

© The Author(s) 2018
M. S. Winchester et al. (eds.), *Global Health Collaboration*, SpringerBriefs
in Public Health, https://doi.org/10.1007/978-3-319-77685-9_3

south, there is the opportunity to access greater resources and capacity from institutions in the global north, and further the reputations of educators in global health related curricula and future practitioners (Adams and Sosin 2016; Bozinoff et al. 2014; Crump and Sugarman 2008; McCoy et al. 2008). For institutions in the global north, engaging in partnerships can lead to an increased understanding of: diseases that may be more prevalent in the global south, diverse social determinants of health, and different care provision and challenges in low-resource settings (Adams and Sosin 2016; McCoy et al. 2008; Provenzano et al. 2010; Stys et al. 2013). Moreover, sequelae from these experiences have indicated an increased student interest to continue work in low-resource settings and public health arenas (Crump and Sugarman 2008; Gupta et al. 1999).

Criticism of short term global health experiences includes concerns regarding lack of knowledge about benefits to institutions and communities hosting northern students; lack of reciprocity with student or faculty exchanges; economic and labor burden to settings hosting northern students; concerns of student engagement beyond their training; lack of language training and sustainability concerns, among others (Aldulaimi and McCurry 2017; Ouma and Dimaras 2013). However, for participants in these programs regardless of where they fall on the north-south divide, there are opportunities to develop and foster intercultural awareness; and exchange knowledge across clinical, medical, public health and health science domains (Inglis et al. 2000).

Most learners on short term global health fieldwork experiences are from the global north and this leads to missed opportunities in partnership building, capacity development, and network building. These cross-cultural exchanges can benefit all participants through improving communication and adaptability to new situations, challenging notions of what global health is or is not, and bringing innovative ideas inspired through international experiences to domestic health efforts. Programs aiming to succeed in these goals must be founded on dialogic principles whereby program planning and curricula development evolve through conjoint discourse and iterative processes between north and south stakeholders. In this chapter, we share two examples in global health education that promote and operationalize bi-directionality in short-term global health exchanges: one conducted at the graduate level and one at the undergraduate level.

3.2 An Approach in Graduate Education

Innovative models in graduate global health education are necessary to address two main challenges in global health international experiences: (1) Learners from the global north often travel to international sites without a good understanding of the context on the ground. (2) Learners from the global south have often been excluded from the opportunity to travel and gain a world perspective related to health systems.

Many opportunities for international field experiences at the graduate level are unstructured and oftentimes students may travel to new environments where they do not have a firm understanding of the local context, challenges, or history. The lack of structured programs for global health interns reflects missed opportunities for both students and partner institutions. Other than financial benefits, or leveraging opportunities of international collaboration, many partnering institutions do not develop precise goals about how the internship would benefit their institution or communities. The roles of these partner institutions may then become relegated to exhibiting a platform of community service, facilitating data collection through identification of sites/participants, providing students with translators and providing necessary managerial and hospitality inputs. Furthermore, weak or no mentoring is accompanied by the danger that students would return from their internship without any additional knowledge. In an alien cultural setting, students risk identifying only what they know, and collecting data on what they believe they know. When reported as publications or presentations, the internship experience would reinforce existing views, defeating the overarching goal of the short-term internship which is to acquire knowledge on health in a different setting. Lack of appropriate partner institution mentoring could also exacerbate global health inequities through reinforcing existing values without an appropriate understanding of the local context.

Partner institutions from the global south also lose an enormous opportunity for furthering global health dialogues. A structured program allows a dissection of the country's public health history, tracing how events in the past, including the colonial past of most nations of the global south have shaped the present health situation. Without a structured course, the achievements and the challenges of developing countries cannot be communicated to students visiting from regions with different socio-economic levels and standards of living. A structured program is imperative for a true discussion of "global" health. It would be essential for identifying new research areas, and breaking the monotony of focusing research activities specifically to issues relating to "unfinished agendas".

Program in India The Field Course on Public Health in India, and the accompanying online courses offered by the School of Health Sciences of Savitribai Phule Pune University (SPPU), emerged from such an argument. The Field Course aims to re-examine the existing "global" narrative on public health in India and the present ideas of public health achievements and capabilities. Globally, the health achievements of India are overshadowed by reports of its poor ranking among countries in terms of its health indicators. These rankings overshadow the fact that the country is in middle of an epidemiological transition and that the average health statistics for different states represent as a baffling range, from indicators similar to sub-Saharan African countries to those indicators that are similar to those of upper middle income countries. Although, this context of "nations within a nation" appears briefly in global literature, it defines the primary challenge facing public health in India.

The Field Course is designed as a rigorous 4 week course with the goal of illustrating the health status of the Indian population, health policies and interventions, and the delivery of public health interventions including local innovations. It also includes the impact of these interventions in terms of achievements, challenges, and the role of different factors in influencing the outcome of interventions. Underlying these goals is the message that while the science of public health is global, its practice and outcomes are shaped by the local context- the people, their socio-cultural, biological, physical, economic, and political environments, and the health policies, services and interventions.

The online course will flatten financial and time-related barriers to global health education between countries. Online training, prior to the country visit, would complement the onsite program developed for students from the global north visiting SPPU. This would help visiting students prepare physically and mentally to face a strange culture and environment. The on-site course is aimed at challenging students to dissect out the proximal and distal determinants that influence the efficiency of the health system in India. The courses also aim at stimulating a problem-solving approach among students.

We believe the success of the program was due to the formal structured curriculum, solid and constant student supervision, and the combination of field visits and classroom exercises. Activities such as field visits gave learners a real picture of the situation, kept learners engaged, and debunked any myths held about India and the public health system. Classroom exercises solidified course material and allowed for time to debrief experiences at the field visits. The program also invited three Indian students to formally attend the program. These students attended all classes, were present for all field visits, and engaged actively in the discussion and assignments. This gave all participants the opportunity to explore cultural context, people, and life in the city.

Program in the United States Pennsylvania State University's (PSU's) Global Health Exchange Program (GHEP) began with a goal to facilitate a global conversation between graduate students across countries and cultures about healthcare systems and models that provide access to care. By exposing graduate students early to diverse approaches to health care access and models of healthcare delivery systems, students gain a broader and more informed global perspective. A global perspective will benefit students throughout their career and may ultimately benefit their own local public health community through bringing a unique perspective and open mind to possible public health solutions.

GHEP invites students from international partner institutions to participate in a public health training course in Hershey, Pennsylvania and sends PSU students to international partner institutions to gain first-hand perspectives on health care challenges and systems in each host country. GHEP's structure is grounded in university linkages that offer structured international programs for PSU students and are interested in sending their students to PSU for a structured program. GHEP aims to prime learners on how to function in a new health system and how to understand the way other health systems work and why. This focus on having learners understand how to assess and approach different health systems was inspired by the 2010 Lancet Commission report that called for an approach that is 'systems based to improve the performance of health systems by adapting core professional competencies to specific contexts, while drawing on global knowledge' (Frenk et al. 2010:1924). This two-way exchange program is based in the global health competencies set forth by the Association of Schools and Programs in Public Health and the Consortium for Universities in Global Health (Ablah et al. 2014; Jogerst et al. 2015).

PSU students are able to complete their required three credit internship through traveling abroad with GHEP. GHEP international partner institutions each offer programs to immerse students in the health system and culture in their country and offer mentored projects suitable to each learner's area of interest or skillset. Before travel, PSU students attend preparatory meetings that cover an overview of the health system and current events in the country where they will complete their internship, health and safety, and cultural humility. Students are required to keep a daily log of reflections and submit a final assignment related to their mentored project.

GHEP's short-term summer training program in the United States (US) provides the opportunity for international students to gain a first-hand look into the US healthcare system. The intensive course includes faculty lectures on US governmental structure and health policy, as well as discussions of current major public health challenges faced by the US. These knowledge-based sessions are supported through site visits to national and state government offices, as well as community organizations working to improve health and advocate for change on a local level. Concurrently, students visit different types of healthcare facilities to gain a better understanding of the levels and options for care in the US. PSU students are also offered the opportunity to attend this course to foster student dialogue in health and make connections for students outside of the US. At the end of the program, students are asked to conduct a presentation in pairs that join students from different countries and compare health challenges and systems in their home countries and the US. In the end, students should come away with a good understanding of the US healthcare system and how it compares across the countries in which we have student representation.

3.3 An Approach in Undergraduate Education

PSU's global health education efforts at the undergraduate level aim to facilitate the expansion of students' interests in global health care provision, access and issues through the offering of a 21–27 credit minor in global health. This program is transdisciplinary – open to majors across the university, and exposes students to theoretical, scientific and practical issues affecting the health of people in various countries and world regions. Comprised of both an academic in-class component and an experiential six-week fieldwork segment, it typically attracts students envisioning careers in medicine, public health, or work in government and non-profit sectors. Through a series of courses students gain understanding of a range of issues that cut across global health domains and competencies promulgated by the Consortium of

Universities for Global Health (CUGH) (Jogerst et al. 2015). These include building knowledge, skills and attitudes across key domains including burden of disease; health and globalization; health determinants; capacity strengthening; promoting collaboration and partnering; ethics; professional practice; and health equity and social justice (Jogerst et al. 2015). In addition, students take a pre-fieldwork course focusing on the culture, health systems and current issues in their fieldwork region; critiques and issues of short-term global health assignments; and psychosocial areas of preparation for this form of immersion experience. Students typically enter the program with little to no clinical care experience. From both an ethical and administrative stance, as well as considerations of risk management, students are taught to understand that their role during the field work segment abroad is as student learners. Within the realm of medical activities, they are observers who shadow and accompany foreign medical professionals and medical students as they undertake hospital and clinic rotations in rural and urban settings.

The field sites in South Africa, Tanzania, and Senegal are forged through official partnerships between PSU and departments in nursing, public health, medicine and other related health disciplines at our partner universities. Formal and transparent relationships between the university and host partners are established through multi-year memoranda of understanding and agreements (MOUs and MOAs). These documents along with consistent email and telephone contact throughout the year, help form partnerships that work together to coordinate student and program logistics from faculty payment to students' short term enrollments in partnering African universities and obtain permissions for student rotations in health and community settings.

An additional level of engagement, targeted to minimize unidirectionality of agency between U.S. and host institutions (Loh et al. 2015) is an annual or bi-annual planning workshop. Sponsored by PSU with costs covered by the program, the weeklong event invites host country faculty coordinators to participate in fieldwork planning, design, implementation and evaluation. With 15–25 PSU students studying across three countries, it is imperative that host partners' perspectives and capacities are understood and privileged. Workshop topics include specific planning and administration reviews, program evaluation and areas of improvement, risk management issues, pedagogical approaches, field site considerations (for example extending or contracting clinical or public health focused rotations), changes in policies, and other areas. Prior to attending, host faculty members are invited to offer academic presentations of their research or work to our university audiences and arrangements are typically made for videoconferencing of presentations.

Program Design and the South African-USA Program As university educators, administrators and healthcare professionals in the field site in South Africa, the participatory and interactive undergraduate program model is an important model to facilitate experiences in global health. At the South African (SA) University, mentors are involved in developing a program schedule determined by areas of interests of the participating students, the visit by the African faculty to USA and most importantly, the local context. The program schedule in the host country is designed to expose students to various aspects of the South African health care system at both health care settings and within the community.

During the 6 week field experience, students are scheduled to participate and interact in the following settings:

1. Hospital/Clinic setting: In this setting, students, students are involved in shadowing health professionals such as doctors and community outreach workers and are exposed to health policy and management. The students gain knowledge and skills as they are exposed to the extent of the burden of disease in SA as well health care practices within the settings.
2. Community setting: In this setting students are exposed to community- based health care workers, old age groups tackling chronic diseases, youth friendly health centers dealing with reproductive health, the private hospital structure, nutrition within private clinics, health-promoting schools, and community projects such as greenery projects. This experience highlights to students the health inequalities, the risk factors, health needs and responses thereof within the society.
3. School Needs Assessment and Project: Toward the end of the field visit, the US students undertake a project in schools (middle to high school levels) in which they conduct a health talk and design health promotion material for learners. The project is based on a needs assessment that they conduct in which they plan and address priority health issues of the school students. Through the project, the undergraduates learn the skills of conducting a needs assessment before designing a health promotion project and health talks based on priority of issues. The program helps to exchange information throughout the 6 weeks and at the end students present their experiences as a presentation to our university faculty, administrators and their medical mentors in the health communities.

In short, the model facilitates the students to gain knowledge and skills on the various aspects of global health (burden of diseases, health care practices, research, health policy and management, primary health care and determinants of health in SA). Some cultural aspects and beliefs within South Africa are explored as these contribute significantly to the health of the people.

For the US program planning component, South African university management provides permission for the faculty to visit the USA based on the Memorandum of understanding (MOU) and the Memorandum of Agreement (MOA).The plans are made well in advance of the proposed period of the activity. Orientation is planned and prepared for participating students at the initial part of the program at the host country. Prior to placement of students to various settings, in-country orientation is conducted for the students around issues of security, transportation, accommodation, social life, the university and surrounding communities. Students are also introduced to the University management and key staff members. This allows students to know the country, be aware of existing health needs and different ways of responding to such needs. The plans are made flexible to accommodate participating student's quest for knowledge and people they would like to meet during the period of their stay.

Program Design and the Senegal-USA Program Perspective The internship in Mbour, Senegal is a great opportunity for students and for the hospital. Indeed, the students find themselves in a context that puts him to the test with the discovery of new global health realities; it requires an open mind and a capacity for adaptation. The field work experience should allow students to gain maturity. The hospital is open to global partnerships and to the benefits derived from networking with other partners. An inter-hospital twinning with Mbour Hospital and a global US partner would be an asset to our development.

The Senegal program culture-centric approach to training students, and developing community-academic partnerships. Daily, students rotate through the main hospital in MBour Senegal, participate in research projects with supervising US and Senegalese faculty and attend local research conferences and events.

The goal is to have students engage in the local culture as a vehicle for understanding local health. To achieve this goal we employ two major strategies. First we partner with a nonprofit organization with sites in the US and Senegal that takes a grassroots, community-based approach to non-communicable disease prevention and management. This organization, allows students to participate in local community health screenings and community health capacity building programming such as diabetes support group meetings and events while in Senegal.

Second, we engage in cultural activities on a weekly basis. The premise of the Senegal site is to learn about health through culture. Students attend athletic events, music events, are hosted for dinner by local families, take Senegalese dance class, attend weddings, visit cultural sites such as Goree Island, shop at local markets and learn the local language. Program leaders from both Senegal and the US have daily discussions with students about how they are interpreting local culture, context and health issues. While ultimately the cultural emersion helps the students gain, students may feel awkward or uncomfortable being an outsider and often need help to process daily experiences.

African Faculty Program Planning USA Meeting Perspective Meeting with the coordinators from the other African countries along with PSU program administrators and faculty provided a critical and important opportunity of discussing face-to-face issues pertaining to the program – the strengths, challenges and further improvements including sustainability. We learn many things from each other. This creates a sense of friendship and ownership of the program. It creates a friendly networking South – South and also South – North kind of close relationship. Automatically, we feel valued and our confidence and motivation in coordinating this program is enhanced again and again.

Conducting in person PSU is an opportune time to familiarize ourselves with the students and make friends with them when they come to the country. It gives them knowledge of our local culture and customs before arriving in the host country. It creates a unique relationship, not as new people when we meet in the country. Their conversation and questions mostly serves to help us know their expectations and make preparations accordingly. It helps allay culture shock and prepares students' adjustment to the foreign culture.

Inter-program exchanges can lead to other benefits such as learning new skills and techniques. Visiting PSU also helps improve my teaching skills and ability to handle students. In addition, it makes the coordinators familiar with resources such as how to teach in the simulation lab. For example, the US simulation lab is of a high standard and from our time visiting it, I learned how to improve our simulation lab in Muhumbili, Tanzania. Future improvements to the USA-African program could benefit from online sessions between Pennsylvania State University and our universities using video – conferencing where the students from each side can learn from each other and familiarize prior to onsite meeting in the countries.

3.4 Conclusion

Efforts in bilateral partnerships in both graduate and undergraduate global health educational programs offer multiple benefits for involved institutions. The benefits reported in the literature include the opportunity to strengthen ethical partnerships, educate the global workforce, empower trainees to be agents of change in their home institutions, and improve training and opportunities at host institutions (Arora et al. 2017). In addition to those advantages, our bidirectional global health programs yield the following rewards including increased interaction between faculty and students in the global north and the global south, strengthened sense of community between institutions, and an improved understanding of diverse health care systems, approaches to health challenges, and cultural values related to health and health care delivery.

Challenges related to our bidirectional global health education programs include funding students and faculty from the global south to travel to the United States for training and creating structured programs that minimize the burden of hosting institutions including orienting students to the local context, logistics, curriculum development, cultural or language barriers, and mentorship (Arora et al. 2017). The time required to host students and ensure a successful visit can be disruptive and burdensome for faculty and staff at host institutions and take away time from regular commitments (Provenzano et al. 2010). Before any educational partnership is established, it is necessary to weigh the benefits of the exchange with the costs of diversion of faculty and staff time (Provenzano et al. 2010). It is also important to communicate with host institutions to establish their needs to run such a program. Additionally, it may be difficult to find ways for students to benefit the host institution and serve the needs of the community in which they visit (Provenzano et al. 2010). Structured and reciprocal educational programs strive to meet these challenges, but can fall short. It can be difficult to identify areas for reciprocal arrangements due to challenges in aligning faculty priorities in terms of the proportion of effort dedicated to teaching and research, educational program goals including necessary competencies and goals students are required to meet through international experiences, as well as institutional priorities in terms of differing university strategic goals and resources available that support educational initiatives. These challenges are difficult to overcome and each institution will have their own approaches to mitigating the challenges. Facilitating early and often communication is critical to finding appropriate solutions to financial, logistical, educational, cultural/language, and mentorship concerns.

The educational programs developed by the SPPU and PSU helped build bilateral relationships between institutions and faculty, educate students about the public health systems in India and the United States, incorporate views of the local experts, and expose students to various dimensions of health challenges in India and the United States. The undergraduate global health educational program through PSU and its partners in Africa offers a model for bidirectional faculty collaboration. Both models for global health education can provide new ideas for global health educational development and partnership.

This chapter describes two distinct methods of strengthening global health educational partnerships and increasing bilateral dialogue between partners at the student and faculty level. Short-term international internships allow for a unique opportunity to support bilateral partnerships in global health education. Further expansion of bilateral global health educational programs is necessary for strengthening international partnerships and building a global health workforce that has a shared experience in global health exchange and bidirectional dialogue.

Challenges
- Identifying opportunities for mutual benefit between institutions is difficult due to potential misalignment in faculty priorities, required competencies for students, as well as possible diverging institutional priorities.
- Students need to be prepared with a good understanding of the local context surrounding public health challenges and initiatives before they travel for international global health opportunities.
- Adequate resources need to be allocated to students and faculty from the global south to participate in domestic and international global health trainings and collaborative meetings

Lessons Learned
- Short term international internships allow for a unique opportunity to support bilateral partnerships in global health education.
- Further expansion of bilateral global health educational programs is necessary for strengthening international partnerships and building a global health workforce that has a shared experience in global health exchange and bidirectional dialogue.

References

Ablah E, Biberman DA, Weist EM et al (2014) Improving global health education: development of a global health competency model. Am J Trop Med Hyg 90(3):560–565. https://doi.org/10.4269/ajtmh.13-0537

Adams LV, Sosin AN (2016) Beyond visas and vaccines: preparing students for domestic and global health engagement. Ann Glob Health 82(6):1056–1063. https://doi.org/10.1016/j.aogh.2016.10.010

Aldulaimi S, McCurry V (2017) Ethical considerations when sending medical trainees abroad for global health experiences. Ann Glob Health 83(2):356–358. https://doi.org/10.1016/j.aogh.2017.03.001

Arora G, Russ C, Batra M et al (2017) Bidirectional exchange in global health: moving toward true global health partnership. Am J Trop Med Hyg 97(1):6–9. https://doi.org/10.4269/ajtmh.16-0982

Bozinoff N, Dorman KP, Kerr D et al (2014) Toward reciprocity: host supervisor perspectives on international medical electives. Med Educ 48(4):397–404. https://doi.org/10.1111/medu.12386

Crump JA, Sugarman J (2008) Ethical considerations for short-term experiences by trainees in global health. JAMA 300(12):1456–1458. https://doi.org/10.1001/jama.300.12.1456

Frenk J, Chen L, Bhutta ZA et al (2010) Health professionals for a new century: transforming education to strengthen health systems in an interdependent world. Lancet 376(9756):1923–1958. https://doi.org/10.1016/S0140-6736(10)61854-5

Gupta AR, Wells CK, Horwitz RI et al (1999) The International Health Program: the fifteen-year experience with Yale University's Internal Medicine Residency Program. Am J Trop Med Hyg 61(6):1019–1023

Inglis A, Rolls C, Kristy S (2000) The impact on attitudes towards cultural difference of participation in a health focused study abroad program. Contemp Nurse 9(3–4):246–255

Jogerst K, Callender B, Adams V et al (2015) Identifying interprofessional global health competencies for 21st-century health professionals. Ann Glob Health 81(2):239–247. https://doi.org/10.1016/j.aogh.2015.03.006

Loh LC, Cherniak W, Dreifuss BA et al (2015) Short term global health experiences and local partnership models: a framework. Glob Health 11(1):50. https://doi.org/10.1186/s12992-015-0135-7

McCoy D, Mwansambo C, Costello A et al (2008) Academic partnerships between rich and poor countries. Lancet 371(9618):1055–1057. https://doi.org/10.1016/S0140-6736(08)60466-3

Ouma BD, Dimaras H (2013) Views from the global south: exploring how student volunteers from the global north can achieve sustainable impact in global health. Glob Health 9(1):32. https://doi.org/10.1186/1744-8603-9-32

Panosian C, Coates TJ (2006) The new medical "missionaries"—grooming the next generation of global health workers. N Engl J Med 354(17):1771–1773. https://doi.org/10.1056/NEJMp068035

Provenzano AM, Graber LK, Elansary M et al (2010) Short-term global health research projects by US medical students: ethical challenges for partnerships. Am J Trop Med Hyg 83(2):211–214. https://doi.org/10.4269/ajtmh.2010.09-0692

Stys D, Hopman W, Carpenter J (2013) What is the value of global health electives during medical school? Med Teach 35(3):209–218. https://doi.org/10.3109/0142159X.2012.731107

Chapter 4
Intercultural Adaptation of the "Secret History" Training: From South Africa to Germany

Eva Hänselmann, Caprice Knapp, Michael Wirsching, and Simone Honikman

4.1 Introduction

Global institutional collaborations are typically focused on research, education, or training. These collaborations provide opportunities for the exchange of information and academic practices across countries and hemispheres. However, in addition to academic purposes, one of the ultimate goals of collaboration should be that local communities benefit from their involvement.

These motivating factors came together in 2016 when the "Secret History" adaptation project was funded by the Pan Institution Network for Global Health (PINGH). The primary aim of the project was to culturally adapt and test a novel training – the "Secret History" method – that supports empathy and self-care skills for health workers.

This chapter describes the project, but also illustrates how this project benefitted from a true global collaboration. The project team included researchers from University of Cape Town, South Africa, where the method was developed; Pennsylvania State University, USA; and the target institution, University of Freiburg Medical Center, Germany. The team brought together extensive knowledge of the intervention, implementation, evaluation, clinical expertise, access to the relevant participants, and international project management.

E. Hänselmann (✉) · M. Wirsching
Clinic for Psychotherapy and Psychosomatic Medicine, Faculty of Medicine and Medical Center, University of Freiburg, Freiburg im Breisgau, Germany
e-mail: eva.claudia.haenselmann@uniklinik-freiburg.de

C. Knapp
Department of Health Policy and Administration, Pennsylvania State University, State College, PA, USA

S. Honikman
Perinatal Mental Health Project, Alan J Flisher Centre for Public Mental Health, Department of Psychiatry and Mental Health, University of Cape Town, Cape Town, South Africa

© The Author(s) 2018
M. S. Winchester et al. (eds.), *Global Health Collaboration*, SpringerBriefs in Public Health, https://doi.org/10.1007/978-3-319-77685-9_4

Being part of PINGH allows for efficient replication in other PINGH member institutions, and institutions beyond PINGH. In this way, the project broadens PINGH's scope of interventions, training, and improvement of clinical care. The experiences and lessons learned from this project not only contribute to the body of scientific knowledge, but allow for reflection and response to the strengths and opportunities of global collaborations.

4.2 "Secret History"

The original setting and rationale Staff working in obstetric services in South Africa are confronted with high levels of obstetric morbidity and mortality, and frequently experience compassion fatigue and burnout (Mashego et al. 2016). Linked to this, there have been several reports over the years of abusive care by healthcare staff of their pregnant clients, especially in the labour ward setting (Jewkes et al. 1998; Kruger and Schoombee 2010; Rothmann et al. 2006; Odhiambo 2011).

At the same time, in South Africa, the diagnostic prevalence of depression during pregnancy and in the first postpartum year, ranges from 22% to 47% and is closely associated with social adversity including food insecurity and domestic and community violence (Rochat et al. 2011; van Heyningen et al. 2016). These rates compare with the 11–12% range typically cited for high income countries (Woody et al. 2017).

The Perinatal Mental Health Project (PMHP), at the University of Cape Town, argues that a critical foundational element to mental health service development for mothers is to address, as an initial step, the distress and abuse so typical in the obstetric environment. In order to do this, the "Secret History" training method was developed in 2004.

The training This 2 to 4 h interactive training session uses group role-play to enable care providers to re-enact a typical disrespectful scenario, and thereafter an empathic engagement between provider and mother (patient). Scenarios are designed to reveal the social and emotional vulnerabilities of both characters. Participants adopt the role of care provider or patient, and with the help of facilitators, elements of the characters' histories are revealed in stages to encourage spontaneous interaction. The roles are reversed for each scenario so that each participant can experience the perspective of "the other." During the simulation of both the disrespectful and empathic cases, the facilitators interrupt the "play" and ask how the characters are feeling and what they need. A didactic component on empathic engagement skills is interposed between the two cases and a debriefing session occurs after each of the cases is enacted. A discussion on self-care is incorporated into each of the debriefing sessions.

The target setting and rationale Major problems in South African (SA) public health settings such as lack of supplies, unsafe working environments and limited support and supervision (Breier et al. 2009; Coovadia et al. 2009), as well as social issues of SA nurses such as economic vulnerability and prevalent domestic violence (Oosthuizen and Ehlers 2007; Sprague et al. 2016), by and large do not apply to German nurses and midwives and their working conditions. However, there are a number of other factors supporting the relevance of the "Secret History" method for the medical field in High Income Countries (HICs).

First, the relevance of empathic care for optimal health outcomes is well known globally. Apart from state-of-the art pharmaceutical and technical treatment, the relationship between the health care provider and the patient is a very powerful tool to ensure patient adherence and satisfaction, both of which are desirable health outcomes (Fuertes et al. 2007; Hillen et al. 2011). In the perinatal period especially, interpersonal quality of care is relevant for prevention (e.g. Ashby et al. 2016; Olds 2006). Empathic care can exert a positive influence on the emotional experience of the mother during pregnancy (Seefat-van Teeffelen et al. 2011) and birth (Moloney and Gair 2015).

Second, obstetric violence is not restricted to health care institutions in Low and Middle Income Countries (LMICs). As a recent review on the issue shows, "verbal abuse of women by health providers during childbirth was commonly reported across all regions and country income levels" (Bohren et al. 2015). Women reported being blamed by health workers for poor health outcomes and not being involved in the decision-making process, while also reporting physical abuse such as being neglected during labour, non-consented procedures, and being denied pain medication (Forssén 2012). Another study reports ineffective communication of providers with women during childbirth (e.g. dismissal of women's concerns during labour, no communication of the need for surgery or intervention) making the women passive participants with only an illusion of choice. Again, participants in the study reported that they felt alone and neglected during their deliveries (Redshaw and Hockley 2010).

Third, the aspect of receiving kind, supportive, and respectful care during labour and birth is known to be of high relevance to women in HICs. While they choose to deliver in a health facility that offers technically sound care to ensure positive health outcomes for themselves and their babies, they also expect emotional support (Bohren et al. 2015). They are dissatisfied when staff appear as inconsiderate or uncaring, and when they were excluded from decision-making—their labour being "taken over by strangers or machines" (Small et al. 2002). In HIC hospital settings, obstetric care is typically oriented to organizational protocols, revolving around routines and standard practices rather than around the women's individual concerns (Coyle et al. 2001). Again, this leads to depersonalized care, lack of rapport between providers and patients, and the perception that health care providers lack empathy (Coyle et al. 2001).

For the German context, no scientific studies on birth experiences in the hospital setting could be found. However, the numerous recent reports (Mundlos 2015) and counselling literature (Sahib 2016; Meissner 2011; Bloemeke 2015) available on the topic show that it is a pressing issue.

When searching for existing trainings in empathy and/or self-care for professionals working in maternal care in a systematic literature review (Hänselmann et al. 2017), 13 final results were retrieved. Of those, only four formats combined empathy and self-care as learning objectives. Moreover, most of the reported training formats were modules in undergraduate or vocational training (12), and only one was designed as further training for practising maternal care staff. Based on these findings, the "Secret History" appears unique. The training is in a flexible and short format. It can be used in vocational and undergraduate contexts, as well as in work-based further training, and brings together the complementary skills of empathy and self-care.

Existing communication training at the University of Freiburg (for medical students), Freiburg Academy of Medical Professions (for midwifery and nursing students), and at the obstetric ward of University of Freiburg Medical Center (work-based further training for practicing nurses and midwives) also takes the form of case-based role-play, involving the participants actively. Usually, role-play is conducted either in small groups of three, where the roles of care provider, patient, and observer are rotated, or in a fish-bowl setting with two participants taking the roles of care provider and patient and the rest of the group functioning as observers. In this setting, desirable communication and empathic behavior is practiced. However, group role-play, as well as the acting out of disrespectful care as an opportunity for further reflection, are not being used. Furthermore, the foci on feelings and needs of the care provider (self-care aspect) and on the contribution of the provider's own emotional "baggage" to a potential vicious circle of disrespect are usually lacking (Personal communication with: head of midwifing school on May 3rd and June 9th 2016; head of nursing school on May 4th 2016; nursing expert in charge of further training on the obstetric ward on Jan. 19th and June 9th 2016; psychologist in charge of communication training for medical students on Jan. 25th 2016; trainer for communication in further training for medical doctors on Feb. 15th 2016).

Based on the described contextual background of obstetric care in HICs, and the lack of comparable training formats for empathy and self-care in the context of health care education in Freiburg, the adaptation of "Secret History" was initially judged to be desirable and promising by the project team. This judgment was later confirmed by the results of the focus group discussion and pilot test.

4.3   Cultural Adaptation of Interventions

Health and Culture   Culture has been defined as a "socially constructed constellation consisting of such things as practices, competencies, ideas, schemas, symbols, values, norms, institutions, goals, constitutive rules, artefacts, and modifications of the physical environment" (Fiske 2002).

This definition can be applied to national cultures, but it can also be used to describe cultural differences within a society such as those between different social classes or professions. Barrera refers to these "smaller and more homogeneous unit[s] of social organization within a larger ethnic population that [are] *bound by shared life experiences*" as "subgroups" (Barrera et al. 2013, emphasis added). The staff at a health care organization can be seen as such a subgroup, being bound by shared work experience as well as institutional practices, norms, rules, and environments (cultural dimensions as identified by Fiske 2002) which are different from those in other institutions. Beyond these differences, the constructs of health may not be the same for each cultural subgroup. Winkelman notes, "Concepts of health and disease differ from culture to culture and even from person to person within a culture" (Winkelman 2013).

Consequently, when adapting trainings for health care workers, besides the most obvious adaptation, i.e. language, accounting for cultural differences is also necessary (Bernal et al. 2009). The modification of interventions to fit the needs of a cultural subgroup will be called "cultural adaptation" in this chapter.

Evidence on Cultural Adaptation The literature search conducted for this chapter showed an alarming research gap with regard to cultural adaptation of trainings for health care staff between countries.

Research has been done on cultural adaptation of prevention interventions for patients, especially with regard to prevention and management of HIV/AIDS (e.g. Dévieux et al. 2004; Wainberg et al. 2007; Wilson and Miller 2003; Wingood and DiClemente 2008) and diabetes (e.g. Barrera et al. 2012; Davis et al. 2011; Hawthorne et al. 2010; Osuna et al. 2011). One publication was found on the cultural adaptation of health services (T-share Team 2012), but this is a practical manual for the development and implementation of new interventions. No studies were identified which deal with evaluating and guiding the cultural adaptation of interventions for health care staff.

Also, most of the available studies have been conducted in the US to adapt prevention interventions for minorities within in the country (Barrera et al. 2012; Davis et al. 2011; Dévieux et al. 2004; Latham et al. 2010; Osuna et al. 2011; Whittemore 2007). Only very few studies discuss cultural adaptations of interventions across countries (Ortega et al. 2012; Kumpfer et al. 2008; Skärstrand et al. 2008; Weichold et al. 2006; Williams et al. 2013; Andree Löfholm et al. 2009); and again, none of these focused on health care workers as a target group. We believe that it would be valuable to generate evidence for this specific group and kind of transfer, prior to planning for larger, more elaborate, multi-centre implementation studies.

In particular, more rigorous scientific studies are needed to validate the process of testing cultural adaptation models and to examine whether the adapted programs really render a better fit to the local needs (Castro et al. 2004). Finally, not only proximal health outcomes, but also measures of reach, adoption by health care providers, engagement and maintenance of effects would be worth evaluating to comprehensively consider intervention impact (Glasgow et al. 1999). As Barrera et al. notes, even if cultural adaptations yield equal health outcomes to the original intervention, they could still show better or worse results with view to participation rates and long-term involvement of participants and stakeholders (Barrera et al. 2013).

However, based on the definition of cultural adaptation and cultural group made above, we found it useful to draw on studies that have conducted intercultural adaptation for a different target population for guidance in the process of adaptation pursued in this pilot project.

Cultural Adaptation of Health Care Interventions Whenever a training method is adapted, there is the risk of loss of effectiveness. On the other hand, the omission of adaptation has similar risks. The debate on cultural adaptation evolves around the two terms: fidelity – "the delivery of a manualized prevention intervention program as prescribed by the program developer" and adaptation – "the modification of program content to accommodate the needs of a specific consumer group" (Castro et al. 2004).

If comprehensive adaptation is located at one end of a continuum, maximum fidelity would be at the other end. For example, if everything about a training program is changed, it will be a new program altogether, and it cannot reasonably be called a version of the original one and yield comparable results. Maximum fidelity however could only be achieved by having the same trainers deliver the training at the same place, with the same level of experience, training exactly the same content. However, in practice, this rarely occurs as the term fidelity has been conceptualized as sticking with the "driving elements of a program" (Berkel et al. 2011) clearly acknowledging the need for some degree of variation. As Castro et al. note, "The primary aim in cultural adaptation is to generate the *culturally equivalent version* [italics by EH] of a model prevention program" (Castro et al. 2004). Therefore, in order to facilitate an *equal* learning opportunity to a new target group, interventions need to be culturally modified. So instead of "do the same to everyone" the aim becomes "achieve the same learning effect for everyone".

It has been shown that, "adoption of transported, international programs should not be done without considering adaptation" since culturally adapted versions are more effective than international adopted programs without adaptations (Hasson et al. 2014). Barrera et al. notes that "culturally enhanced interventions" are more effective than "usual care" since cultural fit boost[s] program appeal, appropriateness, and efficacy (Barrera et al. 2013). Lack of cultural fit "would threaten program efficacy, despite high fidelity in program implementation" (Castro et al. 2004). Researchers suggest to develop "hybrid", "adjustable" interventions which "build in" adaptation to assure cultural relevance and community ownership, while also maximizing fidelity of implementation and program effectiveness (Castro et al. 2004).

But the practical questions of adaptation remain such as what to change, how much, and in what order, to provide that equal learning experience. Fortunately, the risks of compromising program efficacy by too extensive or too little modification can be counteracted by following a well-structured, scientifically robust process of adaptation.

In the last 12 years, stage models of adaptation have emerged which show a considerable degree of congruence (Barrera and Castro 2006; Domenech Rodríguez and Wieling 2005; Kumpfer et al. 2008; McKleroy et al. 2006; Wingood and DiClemente 2008). This, together with the effectiveness of stage-developed cultural adaptations speak in favour of the validity and utility of the staged adaptation models (Barrera et al. 2013).

Combined Stage-Model Barrera et al. (2013) synthesize the evidence on multiple adaptation models and suggest a five-step model of cultural adaptation which integrates the respective processes suggested by several research studies (Barrera and Castro 2006; Kumpfer et al. 2008; McKleroy et al. 2006; Wingood and DiClemente 2008). This approach was identified as the most practicable and applicable and served as a basis of the adaptation process followed in the "Secret History" pilot project:

1. Information Gathering – here differences of the original and new target groups are sought out by literature research and preliminary investigation with regard to (a) participant characteristics, (b) program delivery staff, (c) administrative/community factors, and (d) needs and intervention preferences of the new target group. Additionally, suggestions for additions and improvement to the original intervention are gathered even in this early stage and the target community's capacity to implement the intervention is assessed.
2. Preliminary Adaptation Design – here intervention materials and if necessary intervention activities are adapted in cooperation with local stakeholders.
3. Preliminary Adaptation Test – here local staff are trained to deliver the preliminary version of the adaptation and pilot studies are conducted. Evaluation of these sessions should check for (a) implementation difficulties, (b) difficulties with program content or activities/satisfaction with intervention elements, and (c) suggestions for improvement.
4. Adaptation Refinement – here the intervention is revised further based on the precedent step.
5. Cultural Adaptation Trial – this includes a full trial of the revised intervention to check if the desired effects occurred.

4.4 Applying the Adaptation Steps to "Secret History"

Barrera's five stage adaptation process was used to guide and inform die adaptation of the "Secret History" method from the South African to German context (Fig. 4.1).

Step 1 Information Gathering The main activities in this step of adaptation were review of the adaptation literature, as described in the previous section of this chapter. Literature was searched on empathy in perinatal care and strain on obstetric staff in the context of the global north in order to obtain a first impression if the method would be relevant to the target context. Furthermore, contact was made with the

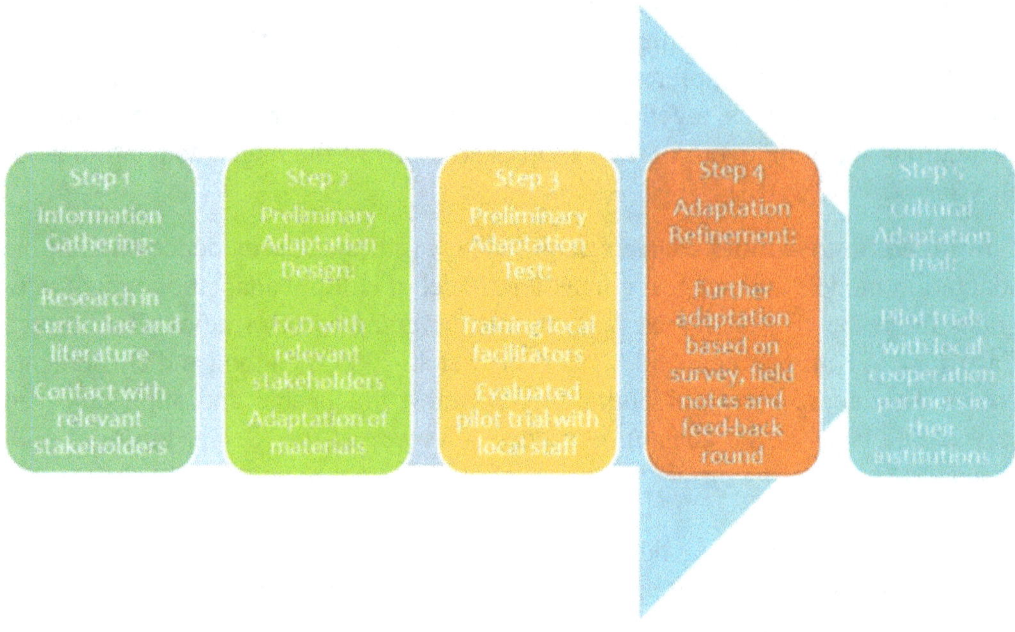

Fig. 4.1 Barrera's steps of adaptation applied to the "Secret History"

relevant stakeholders to find out if they were interested in the method. Stakeholder interest was identified as the main criterion for the target community's capacity to implement the intervention in the context of a university medical center. Stakeholders included experts in mental health care, obstetrics and gynaecology, nursing, and midwifery (Fig. 4.2).

Conversations were aimed to assess interest in the project, feasibility, and sustainability. Stakeholders were also requested to recruit participants for the subsequent activities. Stakeholders were informed about all the possible and intended steps of the project, it was made clear that there was no obligation to participate, and that they could opt out at any stage.

Step 2 Preliminary Adaptation Design Activities in this step include a focus group to find out more about the every-day work setting in obstetrics and about existing and needed education in empathy and self-care. This was used to adapt the training materials. Furthermore, pre and post surveys were developed to be tested in the preliminary adaptation test.

Focus Group
Stakeholders invited staff within their institutions to join the focus group. Along with the invitation and study information, a written consent form was emailed to the participants prior to the discussion. There were two aims of the focus group. First, participants were asked if the "Secret History" training could be of use for the Freiburg obstetrics setting. The second aim was to extract examples of difficulties

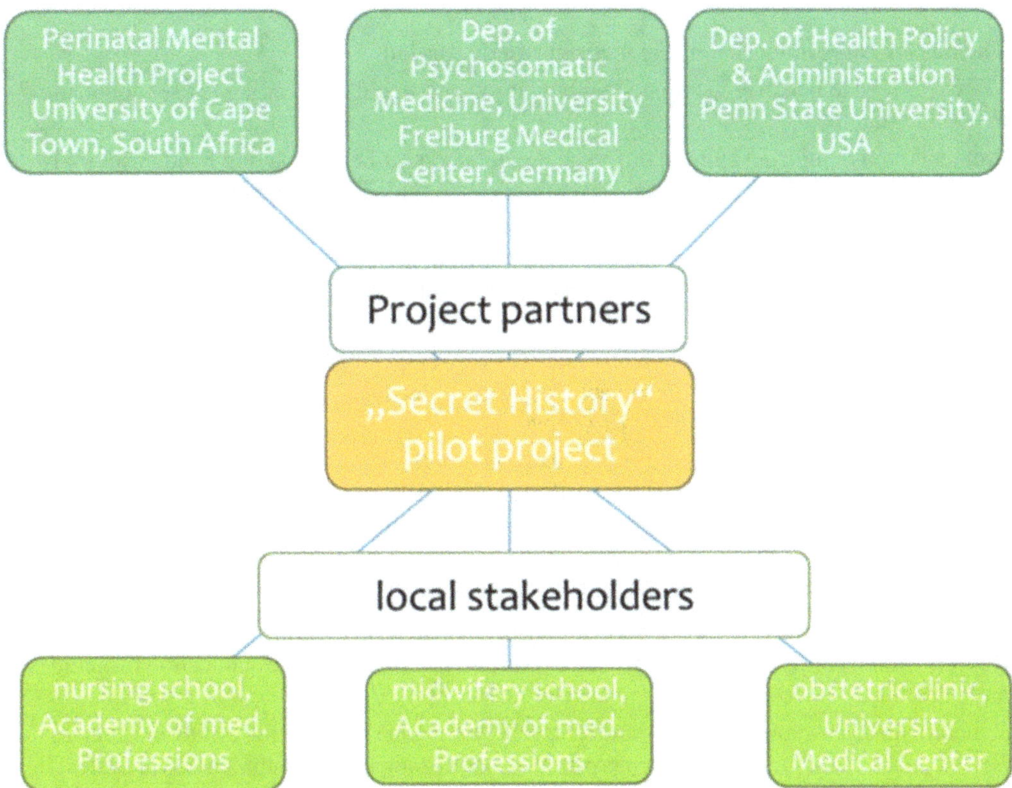

Fig. 4.2 Collaborative network and stakeholders for the "Secret History" pilot project

Freiburg obstetric staff were facing professionally so that the training material could be adapted accordingly and would provide motivation to the participants. Aims were driven by the literature which notes that:

- "sources of non-fit and "mismatch effect," would threaten program efficacy, despite high fidelity in program implementation. Major sources of mismatch are [differences in]: (a) group characteristics, (b) program delivery staff, and (c) administration/community factors" (Castro et al. 2004)
- "[programs may] lack fit and relevance by not addressing significant issues [of the new … group]" (Castro et al. 2004)
- "Community adoption of a program and its local adaptation are enhanced by community ownership or "buy-in" to motivate and sustain local community participation." (Castro et al. 2004)

The focus group included eight participants, lasted two hours and included an introduction and project explanation, structured discussion, and conclusion. Participants filled out a brief demographic survey and were invited to participate in the upcoming pilot testing. The discussion took place in German and was audio-taped. Original versions of the interview guide and the results are available from the first author.

Table 4.1 Focus Group Themes

Themes for cases identified in the focus group discussion
Midwives tend to be "over identified" with their job and find it challenging to "set boundaries" in their commitments.
Problems stemming from cultural differences e.g. fathers-to-be not shaking hands with midwife because of cultural/religious reasons – irritating for the midwife if she doesn't know the background
Communication with the patient: the terms used in obstetric care can be quite fierce and statements like "the baby is too big/too small/in the wrong position" can cause fear in the patient.
Interprofessional communication: hierarchies are very entrenched in the medical center and midwives' experience and knowledge are not always valued and respected by doctors. This is especially problematic in obstetric emergencies.
"Statutory provisions" in the medical field can cause problems. For example, a doctor may instruct a midwife/nurse to carry out procedures which, in a specific situation, may not be in the patient's best interest. This leaves the midwife/nurse in a difficult situation, where the doctor is "safeguarded" against legal action and the midwife/nurse is vulnerable in making a decision to either disobey or do something she believes will not be good for the patient.
Fathers-to-be can be very frightened and can become aggressive towards the nurse/midwife.
Refugee women bring a lot of psychosocial "ballast" and there are communication difficulties and intercultural issues (including female circumcision).
Structural problems: understaffed wards (especially at night), lack of time, midwives/nurses are not well paid, clinics are acting as enterprises (economization of the public medical system)

Adaptation of Materials.

After the focus group was concluded and the data were analysed, emerging themes were used to revise the "Secret History" training materials (Table 4.1). As noted previously, "Secret History" includes two role play exercises and these are based on actual cases, or characteristics of multiple cases, that are common in the local setting.

There was positive feedback from the focus group discussion that it was important to conduct the pilot testing and there was a sense of agency created among local stakeholders through their early and influential involvement in this project.

Survey Development

Finally, evaluation materials were designed to capture the knowledge and attitudes of the participants before and after training as well as the knowledge transfer from the training. Although a few validated tools exist to measure empathy, most are for patients to comment on how empathetic they feel their provider to be. One tool was found for health care providers to self-assess their own empathy; however, the licensing fee for that tool was high and using it would not be sustainable for future studies. Therefore, survey research principles were used to develop the survey, as well as a review of the literature on empathy and self-care. A large item bank was created with the idea that items would be culled after the pilot testing if they exhibited ceiling or floor effects.

Step 3 Preliminary Adaptation Test   Participants were invited via email to join the Train-the-Trainer and Pilot testing of the "Secret History" training five weeks in advance. Invitations were sent to those in a position to be facilitating trainings and practicing or teaching/supervising obstetrics staff; including nurses, physicians, and midwives.

The first aim of the workshop was to train potential trainers for the local pilot sessions. The second aim was to make the method known to local decision makers for further pilot testing and implementation. The third aim was to gather feed-back concerning the quality (or further need) of adaptation of the training. The fourth aim was to test the survey item-bank for further adaptation.

In order to ensure fidelity to the original "Secret History", the developer (S.H.) was asked to facilitate the pilot testing. Given that she does not speak German, a bilingual translator was made available to ensure that the participants could have all the written materials in German. Although all participants were able to speak English, these measures were important as participants of the focus group discussion unanimously stated they may not be able to engage freely in experiential, self-reflective activities in a foreign language. Further to this, a bilingual investigator from the Freiburg team co-facilitated the pilot training.

The Train-the-Trainer and Pilot testing of the "Secret History" training included 13 participants who were mostly female (one male) with extensive job experience (46% of the attendants had more than 20 years of professional experience). Participants included 6 lecturers, 4 practicing nurses/midwives, and 3 other professionals (psychologists, health managers).

The "Secret History" was conducted over four and a half hours. The program included:

- filling out the pre-survey
- introductory ice-breaker
- first role play exercise (disrespectful case)
- break with refreshments
- 1-h didactic session
- second role play exercise (empathic case)
- post survey
- open discussion and feedback on the training program.

Step 4 Adaptation Refinement   In order to maximize feedback from the Train-the-Trainer and Pilot testing, field notes were taken and the role-play and discussion were audiotaped to retrieve participants' comments. Together with the results from the pre and post survey, the feedback yielded the following information which was used to complete the adaptation:

- Although key steps were taken to address the fact that one of the facilitators only spoke English and no negative feedback was noted, we cannot definitively say that there was no impact on the participants. Translation did slow the process and required resources, but this also allowed for the unexpected advantage of facilitators and participants having the time to reflect more thoughtfully on the feelings and needs component within the method. The struggle with trying to articulate the nuances of these through translation allowed for a richer discussion and excavation of the concepts.

- Generally, all participants agreed that the method had a good mix of didactic and learning exercises and that it was relevant for their job. However, the didactic nature of the input on empathic skills did not seem to be as engaging for participants, who had already had a deep knowledge of empathic skills. It was suggested that the didactic part of the course be given in a more interactive way, especially when dealing with such advanced groups of participants. In this way, the training should take in to account the different level of prior training in the group targeted in Germany as compared to the original South African version, thereby addressing possible mismatch-effects (Castro et al. 2004).
- In the survey, 6 participants agreed, 6 were undecided, and 1 disagreed when asked if the cases were typical of the local situation. This disagreement was also voiced in the discussion and the different viewpoints seemed to be connected to the different backgrounds of the participants whereby practitioners in obstetrics tended to agree while trainers and psychologists tended to disagree.
- With respect to the case scenarios used for role-play, several participants suggested in the discussion as well as in the survey, to gather recent problematic situations from the group's own experience rather than using pre-prepared cases. Doing so may improve local effectiveness of the training as cases brought forward by participants would be directly relevant to them. This would more likely result in an optimal cultural fit. Participant involvement in adaptation of training content would enhance the sense of ownership and thus the motivation to participate with the new target group for the intervention (Castro et al. 2004).
- Further suggestions were to give more time for role-play and practice of empathic skills, to conduct the training for interprofessional groups working together in obstetrics (include medical doctors) and to present the method with more detail, so that it could be replicated more easily by participants.
- As only 6 participants said they felt confident they could train others in the "Secret History" method, the objective of training of local staff to deliver the training has not been fully achieved. It seems that several sessions are needed to provide confidence. One major improvement since the time of the pilot testing is that a video illustrating the "Secret History" method is now available online at https://protect-za.mimecast.com/s/37voBeS36N9afa.
- Item analyses of the pre and post test surveys allowed for the revision of the survey instrument. Items with high ceiling or floor effects that did not hang with the domain intended for measurement were culled from the survey. In addition, feedback allowed for revision of items that were unclear or those that the participants felt were not covered by the content.

Overall, the preliminary adaptation test was successful as the program activities were considered highly acceptable by participants. The developer of the training (S.H.) who facilitated the intervention, noted that participants engaged actively and in the manner that was very similar to the original experience in South Africa. For the subsequent cultural adaptation trials, the recommended refinements which were feasible within the restricted time frame and resources were put into practice. These were:

1. Changing the input on empathy and self-care from a didactic to an interactive format
2. Using recent problematic situations from the group's own experience as case narratives rather than using pre-prepared ones.
3. Using a shortened version of the survey to be filled out only after receiving the training.

Step 5 Cultural Adaptation Trials Upon the conclusion of the revisions that were made based on the feedback from the pilot testing, two more training sessions were conducted: one for 22 staff working towards a degree in psychotherapy, facilitated by two people, and another with 12 nursing staff from the women's clinic (oncological ward) facilitated by one person. An effort was made to find other participant groups for these trials apart from the obstetric staff at University of Freiburg Medical Center as a larger follow-up study is planned with this population. Since inquiries made to other midwifery schools in the region were unsuccessful, and time was limited, we elected to use the two options available.

In both cases, the further adaptation proved helpful, leading to a strong involvement of the participants by visibly valuing and integrating their competencies and experience. It seemed to the facilitators that by integrating this amount of interactive generation of course content (cases for role play and empathic skills), the intervention did effectively become a "hybrid" intervention (Castro et al. 2004) with built-in adaptation to assure cultural relevance and community ownership. However, besides the high degree of involvement of the participants, which was observable and positive, there was mixed acceptability of the training in the survey feedback.

A half of the nurses from the women's clinic oncology ward stated that after the training, they were better able to understand their patient's concerns. When asked if the training would affect how they show or feel emotions to their patients, only three agreed. However, a majority of participants agreed, that the training helped them put themselves in their patients' shoes.

The psychotherapy group reported positive feedback about the training. Nineteen out of 22 participants stated that the learning objectives were fully met and 21 participants noted they would be able to use what they learned from the training in their job. As the long-term trainer of the group noted, the special benefit of "Secret History" compared to other trainings is that it shows the participants how their own feelings and needs can contribute to communication problems if these are not addressed.

The different results of the two groups could have been related to the variation in the number of facilitators and the experience of the facilitators. The latter group was facilitated by an experienced practitioner and trainer in psychotherapy together with E.H. who had been working with the method for a longer time and had the opportunity to co-facilitate the Train-the-Trainer and Pilot testing together with S.H, the developer of the method. However, the first group was facilitated by a psychologist who had been exposed to "Secret History" only in the once-off Train-the-Trainer and Pilot testing. Our experience thus confirms Castro et al.'s statement on differences in program delivery staff being one of the major sources of mismatch-effects threatening program efficacy (Castro et al. 2004).

Compared to the pilot test, native speakers conducted both of these trainings in German. Overall, the two trainings demonstrated that the content was fully translated and adapted to the German context. More work is needed to understand how local staff can be optimally trained to facilitate "Secret History" in their institutions and future work will be devoted to this.

4.5   Conclusions

The purpose of this chapter was to describe how a health care worker training program, developed in South Africa, was adapted to the German setting. While the adaptation was multi-staged and conducted over the course of a year, the lessons learned were valuable for future projects. Most adaptations focus on translating content from one language to another. "Translation from one language to another is the most obvious form of program adaptation" (Castro et al. 2004). But reaching cultural equivalence by eliminating sources of cognitive and/or affective non-fit, raises a greater challenge (Geisinger 1994; González et al. 1995). Our experiences made it clear that adaptation is a resource intensive, comprehensive process that can be accomplished in a structured manner following a well-established framework. As Castro et al. note, "two basic forms of adaptation involve modifying *program content* and modifying the *form of program delivery*" (Castro et al. 2004). Our project accomplished both of those and our interdisciplinary team, from three countries, allowed for this to happen in an effective and comprehensive manner. Our project team is encouraged by the positive feedback during this process and the commitment of the academic medical centre to continue to deliver the training. Ultimately, we hope to see the health care worker community in Freiburg sustain the program and to complete adaptation of the "Secret History" training program in other areas.

Challenges
- Adapting instruments across cultural settings comes with barriers of language, translation, time, and context.
- Assessment tools can be prohibitively expensive, particularly in the pilot phases of a project.

Lessons Learned
- Adaptation, although a resource intensive, comprehensive process, can be accomplished in a structured manner following a well-established framework.

- Our interdisciplinary team, from three countries, allowed for complex adaptation of a training to happen in an effective and comprehensive manner.
- Culturally sensitive healthcare worker training has the possibility of improving mental health and empathic care.

References

Andree Löfholm C, Olsson T, Sundell K, Hansson K (2009) Multisystemic therapy with conduct-disordered young people: stability of treatment outcomes two years after intake. Evid Policy 5(4):373–397. https://doi.org/10.1332/174426409X478752

Ashby B, Scott S, Lakatos PP (2016) Infant mental health in prenatal care. Newborn Infant Nurs Rev 16(4):264–268. https://doi.org/10.1053/j.nainr.2016.09.017

Barrera M, Castro FG (2006) A heuristic framework for the cultural adaptation of interventions. Clin Psychol Sci Pract 13(4):311–316. https://doi.org/10.1111/j.1468-2850.2006.00043.x

Barrera M, Toobert D, Strycker L, Osuna D (2012) Effects of acculturation on a culturally adapted diabetes intervention for Latinas. Health Psychol 31(1):51–54. https://doi.org/10.1037/a0025205

Barrera M, Castro FG, Strycker LA, Toobert DJ (2013) Cultural adaptations of behavioral health interventions: a progress report. J Consult Clin Psychol 81(2):196–205. https://doi.org/10.1037/a0027085

Berkel C, Mauricio AM, Schoenfelder E, Sandler IN (2011) Putting the pieces together: an integrated model of program implementation. Prev Sci 12(1):23–33. https://doi.org/10.1007/s11121-010-0186-1

Bernal G, Jiménez-Chafey MI, Domenech Rodríguez MM (2009) Cultural adaptation of treatments: a resource for considering culture in evidence-based practice. Prof Psychol Res Pr 40(4):361–368. https://doi.org/10.1037/a0016401

Bloemeke VJ (2015) Es war eine schwere Geburt: wie schmerzliche Erfahrungen heilen. Kösel, München

Bohren MA, Vogel JP, Hunter EC et al (2015) The mistreatment of women during childbirth in health facilities globally: a mixed-methods systematic review. PLoS Med 12(6):e1001847; discussion e1001847. https://doi.org/10.1371/journal.pmed.1001847

Breier M, Wildschut A, Mgqolozana T (2009) Nursing in a new era: the profession and education of nurses in South Africa. HSRC Press, Cape Town

Castro FG, Barrera M, Martinez CR (2004) The cultural adaptation of prevention interventions: resolving tensions between fidelity and fit. Prev Sci 5(1):41–45

Coovadia H, Jewkes R, Barron P et al (2009) The health and health system of South Africa: historical roots of current public health challenges. Lancet 374(9692):817–834. https://doi.org/10.1016/s0140-6736(09)60951-x

Coyle KL, Hauck Y, Percival P, Kristjanson LJ (2001) Ongoing relationships with a personal focus: mothers' perceptions of birth centre versus hospital care. Midwifery 17(3):171–181. https://doi.org/10.1054/midw.2001.0258

Davis RE, Peterson KE, Rothschild SK, Resnicow K (2011) Pushing the envelope for cultural appropriateness: does evidence support cultural tailoring in type 2 diabetes interventions for Mexican American adults? Diabetes Educ 37(2):227–238. https://doi.org/10.1177/0145721710395329

Dévieux JG, Malow RM, Rosenberg R, Dyer JG (2004) Context and common ground: cultural adaptation of an intervention for minority HIV infected individuals. J Cult Divers 11(2):49–57

Domenech Rodríguez MM, Wieling E (2005) Developing culturally appropriate, evidence-based treatments for interventions with ethnic minority populations. In: Rastogi M, Wieling E (eds) Voices of color: first-person accounts of ethnic minority therapists. SAGE Publications, Thousand Oaks, pp 313–333

Fiske AP (2002) Using individualism and collectivism to compare cultures—a critique of the validity and measurement of the constructs: comment on Oyserman et al. (2002). Psychol Bull 128(1):78–88

Forssén ASK (2012) Lifelong significance of disempowering experiences in prenatal and maternity care: interviews with elderly Swedish women. Qual Health Res 22(11):1535–1546. https://doi.org/10.1177/1049732312449212

Fuertes JN, Mislowack A, Bennett J et al (2007) The physician-patient working alliance. Patient Educ Couns 66(1):29–36. https://doi.org/10.1016/j.pec.2006.09.013

Geisinger KF (1994) Cross-cultural normative assessment: translation and adaptation issues influencing the normative interpretation of assessment instruments. Psychol Assess 6(4):304–312

Glasgow RE, Vogt TM, Boles SM (1999) Evaluating the public health impact of health promotion interventions: the RE-AIM framework. Am J Public Health 89(9):1322–1327

González VM, Stewart A, Ritter PL, Lorig K (1995) Translation and validation of arthritis outcome measures into Spanish. Arthritis Rheum 38(10):1429–1446

Hänselmann E, Husni-Pascha G, Feuchtinger J et al (2017) Training for empathy and/or self-care for professionals and students in maternal care PROSPERO: CRD42017058552. Available from http://www.crd.york.ac.uk/PROSPERO/display_record.asp?ID=CRD42017058552

Hasson H, Sundell K, Beelmann A, von Thiele Schwarz U (2014) Novel programs, international adoptions, or contextual adaptations?: meta-analytical results from German and Swedish intervention research. BMC Health Serv Res 14(Suppl 2):O32. https://doi.org/10.1186/1472-6963-14-S2-O32

Hawthorne K, Robles Y, Cannings-John R, Edwards AGK (2010) Culturally appropriate health education for Type 2 diabetes in ethnic minority groups: a systematic and narrative review of randomized controlled trials. Diabet Med 27(6):613–623. https://doi.org/10.1111/j.1464-5491.2010.02954.x

Hillen MA, de HHCJM, Smets EMA (2011) Cancer patients' trust in their physician-a review. Psychooncology 20(3):227–241. https://doi.org/10.1002/pon.1745

Jewkes R, Abrahams N, Mvo Z (1998) Why do nurses abuse patients? Reflections from South African obstetric services. Soc Sci Med 47(11):1781–1795

Kruger L-M, Schoombee C (2010) The other side of caring: abuse in a South African maternity ward. J Reprod Infant Psychol 28(1):84–101. https://doi.org/10.1080/02646830903294979

Kumpfer KL, Pinyuchon M, Teixeira de Melo A, Whiteside HO (2008) Cultural adaptation process for international dissemination of the strengthening families program. Eval Health Prof 31(2):226–239. https://doi.org/10.1177/0163278708315926

Latham TP, Sales JM, Boyce LS et al (2010) Application of ADAPT-ITT: adapting an evidence-based HIV prevention intervention for incarcerated African American adolescent females. Health Promot Pract 11(3 Suppl):53S–60S. https://doi.org/10.1177/1524839910361433

Mashego T-AB, Nesengani DS, Ntuli T, Wyatt G (2016) Burnout, compassion fatigue and compassion satisfaction among nurses in the context of maternal and perinatal deaths. J Psychol Afr 26(5):469–472. https://doi.org/10.1080/14330237.2016.1219566

McKleroy VS, Galbraith JS, Cummings B et al (2006) Adapting evidence-based behavioral interventions for new settings and target populations. AIDS Educ Prev 18(4 Suppl A):59–73. https://doi.org/10.1521/aeap.2006.18.supp.59

Meissner BR (2011) Emotionale Narben aus Schwangerschaft und Geburt auflösen: Mutter-Kind-Bindungen heilen oder unterstützen – in jedem Alter ; [mit Babyheilbad & Heilgespräch], 1st edn. Meissner, Winterthur

Moloney S, Gair S (2015) Empathy and spiritual care in midwifery practice: contributing to women's enhanced birth experiences. Women Birth 28(4):323–328. https://doi.org/10.1016/j.wombi.2015.04.009

Mundlos C (2015) Gewalt unter der Geburt: Der alltägliche Skandal, 1st edn. Tectum Wissenschaftsverlag, s.l.

Odhiambo A (2011) "Stop making excuses": accountability for maternal health care in South Africa. Human Rights Watch, New York

Olds DL (2006) The nurse-family partnership: an evidence-based preventive intervention. Infant Ment Health J 27(1):5–25. https://doi.org/10.1002/imhj.20077

Oosthuizen M, Ehlers VJ (2007) Factors that may influence south African nurses' decisions to emigrate. Health SA Gesondheid 12(2). https://doi.org/10.4102/hsag.v12i2.246

Ortega E, Giannotta F, Latina D, Ciairano S (2012) Cultural adaptation of the strengthening families program 10–14 to Italian Families. Child & Youth Care Forum 41(2):197–212. Springer, US. https://doi.org/10.1007/s10566-011-9170-6

Osuna D, Barrera M, Strycker LA et al (2011) Methods for the cultural adaptation of a diabetes lifestyle intervention for Latinas: an illustrative project. Health Promot Pract 12(3):341–348. https://doi.org/10.1177/1524839909343279

Redshaw M, Hockley C (2010) Institutional processes and individual responses: women's experiences of care in relation to cesarean birth. Birth 37(2):150–159. https://doi.org/10.1111/j.1523-536X.2010.00395.x

Rochat TJ, Tomlinson M, Bärnighausen T et al (2011) The prevalence and clinical presentation of antenatal depression in rural South Africa. J Affect Disord 135(1–3):362–373. https://doi.org/10.1016/j.jad.2011.08.011

Rothmann S, van der Colff JJ, Rothmann JC (2006) Occupational stress of nurses in South Africa. Curationis 29(2):22–33

Sahib T (2016) Es ist vorbei – ich weiß es nur noch nicht: Bewältigung traumatischer Geburtserfahrungen. Books on Demand, Norderstedt

Seefat-van Teeffelen A, Nieuwenhuijze M, Korstjens I (2011) Women want proactive psychosocial support from midwives during transition to motherhood: a qualitative study. Midwifery 27(1):e122–e127. https://doi.org/10.1016/j.midw.2009.09.006

Skärstrand E, Larsson J, Andréasson S (2008) Cultural adaptation of the strengthening families programme to a Swedish setting. Health Educ J 108(4):287–300. https://doi.org/10.1108/09654280810884179

Small R, Yelland J, Lumley J et al (2002) Immigrant women's views about care during labor and birth: an Australian study of Vietnamese, Turkish, and Filipino women. Birth 29(4):266–277. https://doi.org/10.1046/j.1523-536X.2002.00201.x

Sprague C, Woollett N, Parpart J et al (2016) When nurses are also patients: intimate partner violence and the health system as an enabler of women's health and agency in Johannesburg. Glob Public Health 11(1–2):169–183. https://doi.org/10.1080/17441692.2015.1027248

T-share Team (ed) (2012) Transcultural skills for health and care: standards and guidelines for practice and training. ARACNE, Napoli http://tshare.eu/drupal/sites/default/files/confidencial/WP11_co/MIOLO_TSHARE_216paginas.pdf. Accessed 25 Oct 2017. ISBN 978-88-907245-0-3

van Heyningen T, Myer L, Onah M (2016) Antenatal depression and adversity in urban South Africa. J Affect Disord 203:121–129. https://doi.org/10.1016/j.jad.2016.05.052

Wainberg ML, McKinnon K, Mattos PE et al (2007) A model for adapting evidence-based behavioral interventions to a new culture: HIV prevention for psychiatric patients in Rio de Janeiro, Brazil. AIDS Behav 11(6):872–883. https://doi.org/10.1007/s10461-006-9181-8

Weichold K, Giannotta F, Silbereisen RK et al (2006) Cross-cultural evaluation of a life-skills programme to combat adolescent substance misuse. Sucht 52(4):268–278

Whittemore R (2007) Culturally competent interventions for Hispanic adults with type 2 diabetes: a systematic review. J Transcult Nurs 18(2):157–166. https://doi.org/10.1177/1043659606298615

Williams AB, Wang H, Burgess J et al (2013) Cultural adaptation of an evidence-based nursing intervention to improve medication adherence among people living with HIV/AIDS (PLWHA) in China. Int J Nurs Stud 50(4):487–494. https://doi.org/10.1016/j.ijnurstu.2012.08.018

Wilson BDM, Miller RL (2003) Examining strategies for culturally grounded HIV prevention: a review. AIDS Educ Prev 15(2):184–202

Wingood GM, DiClemente RJ (2008) The ADAPT-ITT model: a novel method of adapting evidence-based HIV interventions. J Acquir Immune Defic Syndr 47(Suppl 1):S40–S46. https://doi.org/10.1097/QAI.0b013e3181605df1

Winkelman M (2013) Culture and health: applying medical anthropology. Jossey-Bass, San Francisco

Woody CA, Ferrari AJ, Siskind DJ et al (2017) A systematic review and meta-regression of the prevalence and incidence of perinatal depression. J Affect Disord 219:86–92. https://doi.org/10.1016/j.jad.2017.05.003

Chapter 5
Provider Workload and Multiple Morbidities in the Caribbean and South Africa

Bilikisu R. Elewonibi, Shalini Pooransingh, Natalie Greaves, Linda Skaal, Tolu Oni, Madhuvanti M. Murphy, T. Alafia Samuels, and Rhonda BeLue

5.1 Introduction

Africa and the Caribbean have the highest prevalence of HIV/AIDS in the world and are also challenged by a chronic non-communicable disease (NCD) epidemic. Although South Africa is an upper- middle income country, and the Caribbean is largely a mix of middle and high income countries, with Haiti the only low income country, their health systems are not fully capable of meeting all the needs of

---

The original version of this chapter was revised. An erratum to this chapter can be found at https://doi.org/10.1007/978-3-319-77685-9_10

B. R. Elewonibi (✉)
Department of Global Health and Population, Harvard T.H.Chan School of Public Health, Boston, MA, USA

S. Pooransingh
Faculty of Medical Sciences, The University of the West Indies, St Augustine, Trinidad and Tobago

N. Greaves · T. A. Samuels
The George Alleyne Chronic Disease Research Centre, The University of the West Indies, Barbados

L. Skaal
Department of Public Health, University of Limpopo, Polokwane, South Africa

T. Oni
Department of Public Health and Family Medicine, University of Cape Town, Cape Town, South Africa

M. M. Murphy
Faculty of Medical Sciences, The University of the West Indies, Barbados

R. BeLue
College for Public Health and Social Justice, Saint Louis Universtiy, St. Louis, MO, USA

patients with comorbidities. In many middle and high-income countries, a dedicated system of care for people living with HIV/AIDS (PLWHAs) was developed in parallel to existing systems of care for chronic NCDs, and these lack an integrated approach. The success of the HIV/AIDS care model has been attributed to increased advocacy, political will, country leadership, empowerment of health workers, increased community involvement and donor funding. These inputs enabled deployment of multi-disciplinary teams, task-shifting, support for adherence via family and community, along with monitoring and evaluation, health system strengthening and continuity of care. Currently, the workload, as well as policies and practices required to manage HIV and NCD care from a patient and health care systems perspective in the Caribbean and South Africa, are not fully known.

This chapter discusses the current state of health care for HIV and NCDs in the Caribbean and South Africa and presents two case studies that examine the challenges faced by patients who need to negotiate these two health care systems for their co-morbid conditions. The cases presented examine the complexity of care for persons living with HIV and Type 2 Diabetes Mellitus (T2DM) living in South Africa and in the Caribbean Islands of Trinidad and Barbados using a modified version of the Cumulative Complexity Model (CCM). This model posits that as the burden of disease and resulting workload increases, the patient capacity to respond to it diminishes.

5.2 Background

5.2.1 HIV and Noncommunicable Disease (NCD) Care in South Africa

South Africa has the largest antiretroviral treatment (ART) program in the world (Dalal et al. 2011; Levitt et al. 2011; Mayosi et al. 2012). As a result of new guidelines for treatment initiation, aggressive intervention and almost full medical coverage have contributed to the progress in prevention of mother-to-child transmission (pMTCT) programs (Johnson 2012; Levitt et al. 2011; Mayosi et al. 2012; World Health Organization 2011). More than 98% of women receive an HIV test during pregnancy and 91.7% of HIV-positive mothers are receiving ART or prophylaxis (Requejo et al. 2012). However, challenges remain, including access to HIV treatment for pregnant women due to stock depletion, further pMTCT due to a lack of feeding support in the postnatal period, and ensuring (Becquet et al. 2009) expansion of treatment to the individuals who still need ART (Mayosi et al. 2012). The program has also struggled with treatment cost, availability of drug suppliers, and sustaining the population (because of logistics in administering medication to a large population, or administration/operation challenges) (Mayosi et al. 2012). There is inadequate data on the long-term consequences of HIV infection and treatment in South Africa. Discrimination and social marginalization continue to be experienced daily by people who are affected by HIV (Mayosi et al. 2012). These social exclusions further contribute to reluctance to test for HIV and to visit dedicated HIV treatment sites.

Most patients in South Africa with NCDs are managed at the primary health care level (Levitt et al. 2011). Major weaknesses of the current structure center around continuity of care, comprehensive care, consistent drug supply, and regular auditing of quality of care (Dalal et al. 2011; Dawson et al. 2013; Levitt et al. 2011; Oti 2013). Support from community health workers for patients with NCDs at the primary care level is rarely available; there is seldom opportunity for patient education, and health workers lack communication skills, which results in suboptimal patient-centered care (Levitt et al. 2011). In addition, there are shortages of essential drugs, lack of access to other drugs, budget constraints that prevent health providers from ordering essential tests, lack of recall systems for non-attenders, and inadequate patient records (Levitt 2008; Levitt et al. 2011). Consequently, patients with NCDs who attend primary care services seldom achieve an adequate level of care.

5.2.2 HIV Care in the Caribbean

In 2004, Trinidad and Tobago (TT) established a National AIDS Coordination Committee (NACC) to coordinate and monitor implementation of the national strategic plan for HIV/AIDS (Duke et al. 2010). The Ministry's National AIDS Programme was renamed the HIV and AIDS Coordinating Unit (HACU) in 2006. One of the priorities for TT was to expand access to HIV testing and in 2006, the Ministry of Health established a same-visit HIV testing program (Laptiste et al. 2013). This program provides confidential testing that confidential testing that does not require laboratory confirmation, providing clients with HIV status information in a single visit. Another successful program is the Rap Port, a youth drop-in center targeting the age group 13–25 years. It was created in response to the epidemic of HIV/AIDS/STIs affecting this population. Its goal was to prompt healthy lifestyle practices by creating a supportive environment (Laptiste et al. 2013). Additionally, the government's prevention of mother-to-child transmission (PMTCT) program was implemented in 1999 in Tobago and 2000 in Trinidad (Laptiste et al. 2013). By 2009, approximately 96.7% of all women attending public antenatal clinics throughout Trinidad and Tobago participated in the program (Laptiste et al. 2013). In 2008, dried blood spot testing for infants was introduced. Antiretroviral therapy is available free of charge at government hospitals and at seven locations throughout the country (Laptiste et al. 2013).

In Barbados, the government provides comprehensive health care, free at the point of delivery, to all its citizens. With the availability of highly active antiretroviral therapy (HAART) since 2002 and the provision of free care and treatment to all HIV-infected persons in Barbados, there has been a consistent decline in the HIV-specific death rate (Kumar et al. 2006, 2007). All HIV-infected persons receive their inpatient care at Queen Elizabeth Hospital and ambulatory care is provided by a centralized HIV clinic that has operated from Ladymeade Reference Unit since 2002 (Kumar et al. 2006). The Ladymeade Reference Unit was established as part of the Government's expanded response to the HIV epidemic and consists of a clinic, in-house pharmacy and an internationally accredited laboratory (Kumar et al. 2006;

Landis et al. 2013). Queen Elizabeth Hospital is the only public hospital in Barbados, providing more than 95% of all inpatient care to the population (Kumar et al. 2007). Barbados also has a well-organized Pediatric HIV Surveillance Program that monitors mother-to-child HIV transmission (Kumar et al. 2004; Kumar and Bent 2003). Since 1990, voluntary antenatal HIV screening, and pre- and post-test counseling has been offered to all pregnant women irrespective of previously known HIV antibody status (Kumar and Bent 2003). Despite easy availability of treatment and care, late presentation has been a major cause of concern (Kilaru et al. 2004, p 4) and widespread stigma and discrimination may be an important issue underlying this problem (Rutledge and Abell 2005).

5.2.3 Non-communicable Disease (NCD) in the Caribbean

The small island developing states (SIDS) in the Caribbean islands face significant challenges with the worst NCD epidemic in the region of the Americas. Premature mortality from NCDs is double the rate in North America. This is due to high prevalence of risk factors, especially obesity, and the limited resources available to address and implement NCD policies (Boda 2013). For example, in Trinidad and Tobago 78% of deaths are due to NCDs, yet there are only 8 physicians per 10,000 people [compared to 25 per 10,000 in the U.S. (Boda 2013)]. These numbers illustrate the reality of the health services strain and area major barrier within Trinidad and Tobago. There are NCD interventions in place, such as the Chronic Disease Assistance Programme (CDAP) supported by Trinidad and Tobago's Ministry of Health. CDAP provides free prescription drugs and other pharmaceutical items to individuals who suffer from diabetes, high blood pressure, cardiac diseases, among other conditions (Ramrattan 2011). However, programs like CDAP do not address the need for NCD prevention.

Heads of government of the Caribbean community (CARICOM) convened in a summit dedicated to NCDs in 2007 (Hospedales et al. 2011). Their declaration, entitled 'Uniting to Stop the Epidemic of Chronic Non-communicable Diseases' (also referred to as the Port of Spain Declaration), focused on prevention and control of NCDs through comprehensive and integrated prevention and control strategies. Each head of government gave clear policy directions for an intersectoral approach that addresses many key risk factors. As Table 5.1 illustrates, Jamaica fully implemented 17 of the 26 tasks set by the 2007 Port of Spain Declaration in 2010 (Samuels et al. 2014). Included in this progress is Jamaica's National Health Fund (NHF), an effort which subsidizes screening and prevention programs targeted at NCDs (established in 2003).

It is clear that there is more work to be done in the area of NCD prevention and control; however, CARICOM's efforts demonstrate hope for regional cooperation and collaboration against the NCD epidemic. These efforts also allow for countries to learn from each other's successes and areas of concern.

Table 5.1 Compliance with 26 indicators from the Port-of-Spain

Highest compliers		
Barbados	20	77%
Trinidad and Tobago	19	73%
Jamaica	18	69%
Bahamas	17	65%
Middle compliers		
Grenada, Cayman Islands, Guyana, St. Lucia	15	58%
Suriname, Antigua & Barbuda	14	54%
Bermuda	12	46%
British Virgin Islands, Dominica	11	42%
Belize	9	35%
St. Kitts and Nevis	8	31%
St. Vincent and the Grenadines	7	27%
Lowest compliers		
Anguilla	5	19%
Turks and Caicos	2	8%
Montserrat	2	8%
Haiti	1	4%

Declaration for CARICOM Countries 2014 score

5.3 Case Studies Examining Patient Challenges Associated with Multiple Morbidity

The case studies presented from South Africa and the Caribbean used a qualitative approach to explore and examine the perspectives and experiences of patients related to workload associated with, and capacity required to manage, HIV/NCD co-morbidity as they negotiate parallel systems of healthcare for HIV and for T2DM. Managing comorbid conditions requires considerable time, effort and money, which add distress to patients who are already burdened by their illnesses. A novel theoretical framework, Shippee's Cumulative Complexity Model, was used to explore how individuals cope with these demands. Phase one of the study was conducted in South Africa and then replicated in the Caribbean, which allowed us to understand workload related to HIV/NCD comorbidity across countries and regions with various income levels, stages of urbanization and health care systems.

5.4 The Cumulative Complexity Model (CCM)

The Cumulative Complexity Model outlines relations between the work delegated by healthcare systems to patients (their burden of treatment), and the ways in which they can balance these burdens with capacity to meet the demands of delegated work. It seeks to summarize the effects of social and clinical factors on patient outcomes

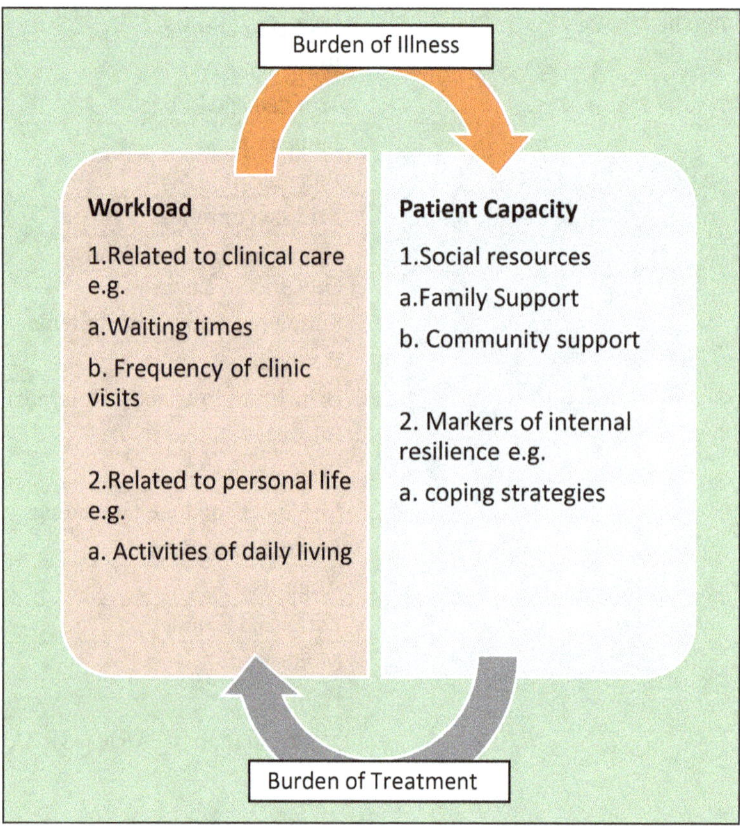

Fig. 5.1 Modified Shippee's Cumulative Complexity Model used in this study on workload in HIV/2TDM

(Shippee et al. 2012). It articulates that a patient's clinical outcomes are influenced by the interaction between two parameters: workload and patient capacity. In the CCM, *workload* refers to those factors which place a demand on a patient's "time and energy", e.g. employment and self-care activities, while *patient capacity* relates to the patient's ability to "handle work". Importantly, patient capacity includes social capital measures such as financial and social resources as well as physical domains such as functional morbidity (Shippee et al. 2012). It is important to note that the CCM is dynamic with complexity of care being driven not only by the primary interaction between workload and patient capacity but also by external drivers of the burden associated with illness and treatment. The domains examined in this study are represented in the modified Shippee's model shown in Fig. 5.1.

5.5 Methodology

5.5.1 Data

Data for these studies were collected through in-person interviews. Constructs explored reflected the proposed theoretical model on cumulative complexity. Specifically, interviews included questions on (i) workload: the demands on patient's time and energy, the demands of treatment, self-care, other comorbidities, access to care for HIV and T2DM treatment, employment status, and family responsibilities and (ii) concerns about the capacity to cope with the workload: financial and social resources, health literacy and morbidity as it affects ability to function. The audiotaped interviews were transcribed verbatim. Random samples of translations in South Africa were periodically checked for accuracy by a third party within the research team. In South Africa, interviews were conducted in English or a local language by a native speaker and then translated back into English for analysis. In the Caribbean, all interviews were conducted in English.

5.5.2 Setting and Sample Size

In South Africa, the study was conducted in two settings. In the Western Cape, the study was conducted in Khayelitsha, a predominantly black African, peri-urban largely informal settlement in Cape Town. The area is largely made up of Xhosa speaking community with about two-thirds of the community employed but live in low-income households. In the Limpopo province, the study was conducted in the Mankweng district, a rural province in South Africa. Most people in Mankweng district are Sotho. Mankweng is made up of peri-urban townships, tribal villages and informal settlements, where large families are living in deprivation, lacking satisfactory water supply, sanitation and adequate access to basic services (Ellison et al. 1996; Statistics South Africa 2014). A total of 10 persons living with multiple morbidity were recruited in Cape Town and 11 in Limpopo.

The Caribbean case study took place in Barbados and in Trinidad and Tobago. Barbados has a population of approximately 280,000 persons, predominantly of the African diaspora; Trinidad and Tobago has a population of approximately 1.4 million persons with two ethnic groups predominating – persons of the East Indian diaspora and those of the African diaspora. Both settings in this case study were urban due to the location of the clinics. This resulted in 20 participants being interviewed in the Caribbean: 10 in Trinidad and 10 in Barbados.

5.5.3 Measures

Multi-morbidity was defined as HIV plus diagnosed T2DM, although many patients likely have additional co-morbidities. T2DM has been selected as the core NCD comorbid condition due to the complexity of its self-management. Eligible patients included those who have initiated ART and have co-morbid diabetes, in the age range of 35–65 years, as this constitutes the group with the greatest number of people who have diabetes and HIV/AIDS. Participants were recruited at the HIV clinics and approached for informed consent to participate. Participants with varied adherence histories (i.e. regular and non-regular attendees) were included. Diagnosed conditions were verified by medical record review after consent was given.

5.6   Data Analysis

The data analysis team was made up of researchers from each research site. Data analysis was done using an iterative process beginning during the data collection phase. Condensed text was abstracted into increasingly higher order headings, creating codes, categories and themes. Qualitative software was used to organize and manage the data analysis. A coding scheme was developed by the research team. Each transcript was coded by one researcher, and then a second researcher independently coded for each researcher's first two transcripts to ensure coding reliability across the team (in South Africa). An analysis group determined the emerging themes from the data.

5.6.1   *Results from Case Study 1: Patient Workload and Capacity for Managing HIV/T2DM in Cape Town and Limpopo*

Perceived Patient Workload Patient workload from managing two chronic, relapsing illnesses emerged as a main theme among participants. Patients felt that they had disease management related workload from both negotiating the healthcare system and *actual* self-care. Patients reported that they experienced clinic-related workload including barriers related to access to care. For example, patients had to negotiate two separate clinics for HIV and T2DM. They also experienced long waiting periods and shortages of healthcare workers, most notably at the diabetes clinic. Self-care related workloads included adherence to nutritional requirements for both conditions, pill burden, engaging in physical activity, ensuring personal safety and dealing with stigma, especially for the HIV diagnosis.

Patient Capacity Patient capacity emerged as a common theme, which included both enablers and challenges to managing diabetes and HIV. Factors related to patient capacity included having a positive attitude about treatment and outcomes, having confidence in medical treatment, having support from family, having strong beliefs in religious or cultural practices, having a reasonable level of health literacy and having financial social support from their family and clinic staff.

Health System There is lack of capacity to provide drugs by the clinics or hospitals due to inventory shortages. The health system is overloaded with chronic patient admissions and frequent visits. Additionally, the health system needs skilled health care practitioners who understand dual drug interactions and side effects so they can communicate these to patients, thereby avoiding late reporting of side-effects and/ or medication noncompliance. Among the challenges cited were the attitude of health care practitioners and the tendency of rural patients to seek services of traditional healers and prophets before presenting at primary health care institutions.

5.6.2 Results from Case Study 2: Patient Workload and Capacity for Managing HIV/T2DM in Barbados and Trinidad & Tobago

The three themes which were found to predominate in this setting are described below. Emerging themes were similar in both sites.

Heath Service Provision Relating to the category of "patient workload of demands", non-personal factors such as the processes involved in heath service provision (e.g. wait times) were found to affect a person's ability to manage their illness and non-illness related tasks more so than family and self-care demands. Patients who require blood tests need to arrive at the clinics early since blood tests are only available for a limited period in the day and for those with an appointment later in the day, this would mean being at the clinic all day. For employed patients attending weekday clinics, this could result in lost wages; an evening or a Saturday clinic would be more accessible and economical for this group, but is not currently available.

Privacy and Dignity Patients with a diagnosis of HIV attending appointments for diabetes management expressed concerns around confidentiality of their medical information. They also indicated that ideally, patients should not be able to see the other patients who attend the dedicated HIV clinic in order to keep their diagnosis private and confidential.

Self-Care and Stigma HIV was considered easier to manage than diabetes. Diabetes management was viewed as much more time intensive with meal preparation time, need for a special diet, exercise, medication and blood glucose testing all being part of the care plan, which makes adherence to a management plan more complex and at times more fearful. Comparatively, HIV management was considered straightforward — "take your meds and go." However, for HIV, there was more discussion around capacity to cope, which was intertwined with experiences of stigma and discrimination. HIV was perceived to present less physical distress or "non-psychological" challenges, but higher mental/emotional challenges compared to diabetes, due to stigma associated with HIV. Diabetes, on the other hand, presented more physical/non-psychological challenges related to disease management as it impacted quality of life, but fewer mental/emotional challenges. Priority areas around diabetes care centred on managing the illness; for HIV the main concerns were related to social determinants (e.g. housing issues, employment, food insecurity), which are linked to stigma and discrimination.

As previously stated, HIV services in Barbados are centralized in a vertical programme capable of addressing the non-HIV chronic care needs of clients, while in Trinidad services are decentralized throughout the clinic system (in addition to a centralised HIV clinic). Interestingly, in Barbados it seems that while episodes of discrimination have been associated with a centralised treatment system, patient preference is for centralised care. In Trinidad and Tobago, participants also preferred a centralized location for their services. All participants desired institutions offering HIV services to take a holistic approach to treatment.

5.7 Discussion

Although the case studies were carried out in separate regions with different socio-demographic characteristics, common themes emerged. The main theme was that health service provision does not adequately cater to patients with HIV and multiple morbidities. Although this health system setup is fairly common, it subjects a person with HIV to community scrutiny, leading to adverse psychological impact (or emotional distress, or feelings of shame and isolation – not sure how specific the data is). A unique theme was observed in the second case study whereby a positive attitude, strong religious beliefs, family support and a reasonable level of health literacy led to adjustment over time. This theme was not present in the first case study.

5.8 Lessons Learned from Cross National Work

This work was an example of successful cross country, cross region collaboration made possible through the Pan Institution Network for Global Health (PINGH). Collaboration resulted in a successful grant application among Institutions of the Network, which made the Caribbean leg of the study possible. Further, cross country collaboration resulted in the sharing of study protocols and expertise in data analysis which, in 2016, culminated in two successful pilot studies. These were used to design the Institutional Review Board proposals used across the research sites in the Caribbean. While there were no challenges in adapting the protocol to a culturally appropriate Caribbean format, the IRB process in Jamaica was not completed in time for their inclusion (or participation). Inter-island collaboration was effected through online meetings and with face-to-face project sensitization and analysis workshops. The face-to-face meetings of the research team were vital quality assurance steps and served to foster cohesiveness. The success of this collaboration was also influenced by the effective leadership of the Network.

5.9 Implication for the Field and Future Work

The HIV programs in developing countries take a 'vertical' approach, with single-disease prevention and treatment programs implemented by specialized health delivery services separate from routinely operated primary health care facilities.

It is characterized by the use of additional and separate staff, registration processes, and newly constructed buildings. However, patient response and health outcomes demonstrate that a model which is patient-centered rather than disease-centered is the only truly sustainable option. To address multiple health challenges simultaneously will require an expansion of health system capacity, particularly in middle- and high-income countries with economically disadvantaged subpopulations. However, existing intervention priorities of HIV/AIDS programs can be accurately applied to NCD care management and a redesign of chronic care systems. Such a coordinated or integrated approach ensures that resources are shared and maximized, bringing an overall improvement to the health system.

This study shows that increasing a patient's psychological capacity as marked by their internal resilience is fundamental to the ability to cope with dual diseases, especially when social, family and community support are diminished as a result of stigma and discrimination. It emphasizes the need for holistic approaches to chronic disease clinical care while advocating for acceptance and normalization of conditions such as HIV in the wider society.

Challenges
- Working across multiple sites requires careful timing and more resources than single-sited work. This may require a staggered study design, rather than concurrent.
- Health system capacities in low and middle income settings are limited by workload and stockouts, making implementation of recommendations difficult.

Lessons Learned
- Cross continental study sites allowed us to understand workload related to HIV/NCD comorbidity in countries with various income levels, stages of urbanization and health care systems.
- Cross country collaboration resulted in the sharing of study protocols and expertise in data analysis resulting in two successful pilot studies being accomplished in 2016.

References

Becquet R, Bland R, Leroy V et al (2009) Duration, pattern of breastfeeding and postnatal transmission of HIV: pooled analysis of individual data from west and south African cohorts. PLoS ONE 4(10):e7397. https://doi.org/10.1371/journal.pone.0007397

Boda PJ (2013) The challenge of combatting non-communicable diseases in Trinidad: access to hospital care. Health 5(11):12

Dalal S, Beunza JJ, Volmink J et al (2011) Non-communicable diseases in sub-Saharan Africa: what we know now. Int J Epidemiol 40(4):885–901. https://doi.org/10.1093/ije/dyr050

Dawson R, Rom WN, Dheda K, Bateman ED (2013) The new epidemic of non-communicable disease in people living with the human immunodeficiency virus. Public Health Action 3(1): 4–6. https://doi.org/10.5588/pha.12.0048

Duke V, Samiel S, Musa D et al (2010) Same-visit HIV testing in Trinidad and Tobago. BMC Public Health 10(1):185. https://doi.org/10.1186/1471-2458-10-185

Ellison GT, De Wet T, IJsselmuiden CB, Richter LM (1996) Desegregating health statistics and health research in South Africa. S Afr Med J 86(10):1257–1262

Hospedales CJ, Samuels TA, Cummings R et al (2011) Raising the priority of chronic noncommunicable diseases in the Caribbean. Rev Panam Salud Publica 30(4):393–400. https://doi.org/10.1590/S1020-49892011001000014

Johnson LF (2012) Access to antiretroviral treatment in South Africa, 2004–2011. South Afr J HIV Med 13(1.) http://www.ajol.info/index.php/sajhivm/article/view/77233. Accessed 25 Oct 2017

Kilaru KR, Kumar A, Sippy N (2004) CD4 cell counts in adults with newly diagnosed HIV infection in Barbados. Rev Panam Salud Publica 16(5):302–307. https://doi.org/10.1590/S1020-49892004001100002

Kumar A, Bent V (2003) Characteristics of HIV-infected childbearing women in Barbados. Rev Panam Salud Publica 13(1):1–9. https://doi.org/10.1590/S1020-49892003000100001

Kumar A, Rocheste E, Gibson M et al (2004) Antenatal voluntary counseling and testing for HIV in Barbados: success and barriers to implementation. Rev Panam Salud Publica 15(4):242–248. https://doi.org/10.1590/S1020-49892004000400004

Kumar A, Kilaru KR, Forde S, Roach TC (2006) Changing HIV infection–related mortality rate and causes of death among persons with HIV infection before and after the introduction of highly active antiretroviral therapy analysis of all HIV-related deaths in Barbados, 1997-2005. J Int Assoc Phys AIDS Care 5(3):109–114. https://doi.org/10.1177/1545109706288587

Kumar A, Kilaru KR, Sandiford S, Forde S (2007) Trends in the HIV related hospital admissions in the HAART era in Barbados, 2004–2006. AIDS Res Ther 4(1):4. https://doi.org/10.1186/1742-6405-4-4

Landis RC, Branch-Beckles SL, Crichlow S et al (2013) Ten year trends in community HIV viral load in Barbados: implications for treatment as prevention. PLoS One 8(3):e58590. https://doi.org/10.1371/journal.pone.0058590

Laptiste C, Beharry V, Edwards-Wescott P (2013) A review of the response to HIV/AIDS in Trinidad and Tobago: 1983–2010. SAHARA J 10(2):72–82. https://doi.org/10.1080/17290376.2013.869406

Levitt NS (2008) Diabetes in Africa: epidemiology, management and healthcare challenges. Heart 94(11):1376–1382. https://doi.org/10.1136/hrt.2008.147306

Levitt NS, Steyn K, Dave J, Bradshaw D (2011) Chronic noncommunicable diseases and HIV-AIDS on a collision course: relevance for health care delivery, particularly in low-resource settings—insights from South Africa. Am J Clin Nutr 94(6):1690S–1696S. https://doi.org/10.3945/ajcn.111.019075

Mayosi BM, Lawn JE, van Niekerk A et al (2012) Health in South Africa: changes and challenges since 2009. Lancet 380(9858):2029–2043. https://doi.org/10.1016/S0140-6736(12)61814-5

Oti SO (2013) HIV and noncommunicable diseases: a case for health system building. Curr Opin HIV AIDS 8(1):65–69. https://doi.org/10.1097/COH.0b013e32835b8088

Ramrattan D (2011) A preventative approach to healthcare (chronic non-communicable diseases) in Trinidad and Tobago. WJSTSD 8(4):339–359

Requejo J, Bryce J, Victora C (2012) Countdown to 2015 maternal, newborn and child survival: building a future for women and children: the 2012 report. In Countdown to 2015 maternal, newborn and child survival: building a future for women and children: the 2012 report (pp. 56–56)

Rutledge SE, Abell N (2005) Awareness, acceptance, and action: an emerging framework for understanding AIDS stigmatizing attitudes among community leaders in Barbados. AIDS Patient Care STDs 19(3):186–199. https://doi.org/10.1089/apc.2005.19.186

Samuels TA, Kirton J, Guebert J (2014) Monitoring compliance with high-level commitments in health: the case of the CARICOM Summit on chronic non-communicable diseases/Controler le respect des engagements de haut niveau en matiere de sante: le cas du Sommet de la CARICOM sur les maladies chroniques non transmissibles. Bull World Health Organ 92(4):270–277

Shippee ND, Shah ND, May CR et al (2012) Cumulative complexity: a functional, patient-centered model of patient complexity can improve research and practice. J Clin Epidemiol 65(10): 1041–1051. https://doi.org/10.1016/j.jclinepi.2012.05.005

Statistics South Africa. (2014). Statistics South Africa (2014): provincial profile Limpopo. Census 2011

World Health Organization (2011) Progress report 2011: global HIV/AIDS response. WHO, Geneva

Chapter 6
Project Redemption: Conducting Research with Informal Workers in New York City

Mallika Bose, Caprice Knapp, Margaret S. Winchester, Agustina Besada, and Amelia Browning

6.1 Introduction and Background

In every country there are workers who perform jobs every day that many citizens do not want to perform. Housekeepers, garbage collectors, and manual laborers are examples of some of these jobs and oftentimes they are done as informal work, meaning they are not part of the formal labor market. In some countries these jobs are done by immigrants or others, such as people with addictions, mental illness, or felons, or those who otherwise find themselves unable to enter the formal labor market (Medina 2008). The establishment of the informal sector provides individuals unable to obtain other forms of formal employment with a way to make a living, which serves as a means to informally reduce unemployment (Afon 2007). Regardless of who is engaged in informal work, these positions are vital to the economy and are typically undervalued and overlooked (Scheinberg and Anschtz 2006).

Informal workers are not typically covered under federal or state legislation protecting worker's rights. Some sub-groups of informal workers, such as manual laborers in the United States and Mexico have formed their own organizations that support their needs as informal workers (Sarmiento et al. 2016). The creation of such groups for U.S. manual day workers (e.g. informal construction workers) arose from the worker's similar cultural and migration identities, and eventually the

M. Bose (✉)
Department of Landscape Architecture, Pennsylvania State University,
University Park, PA, USA
e-mail: mub13@psu.edu

C. Knapp · M. S. Winchester · A. Browning
Department of Health Policy and Administration, Pennsylvania State University,
University Park, PA, USA

A. Besada
Sure We Can, Brooklyn, NY, USA

workers' self-organization garnered support from local communities and organizations (Sarmiento et al. 2016). Informal workers, however, are not unaffected by laws and regulations. For instance, informal workers known as wastepickers can capitalize on state laws in the U.S. that pay people to recycle cans and bottles. For the U.S. wastepicker, laws like the Bottle Bill have aided in the development of the informal sector.

In the case of 'wastepickers', these workers are also important for the environment and contribute to sustainability. Wastepickers, otherwise known as trashpickers, ragpickers, informal recyclers, canners, or scavengers, are people who collect recyclable materials and redeem these for money. In the 1970s, environmental interest groups in the U.S. lobbied for the passage of a federal redemption law, which would have provided monetary incentives for people to collect bottles and cans all over the country (Fiske 1983). The federal legislation did not pass, but over a little more than a decade ago, ten states and Guam passed similar redemption laws (Fiske 1983; BottleBill.org 2016). The purpose of redemption legislation was to provide people with an incentive to act in an environment-friendly way, and while redemption laws have had the intended effect, they also serve as a form of self-employment and economic opportunity for some people. In 2002, Hawaii became the 10th state to enact a redemption law (BottleBill.org 2015).

In India, there are formal and informal wastepickers. Formal wastepickers, such as those in Pune, work with the government as part of the city's recycling program (Chikarmane and Narayan 2000). Pune wastepickers collect all types of potentially recyclable waste from households, sort the waste at designated stations, and the waste is then recycled by the city. Wastepickers in Pune are paid for their duties and they have an organized union. In Nicaragua wastepickers live in landfills (Hartmann 2013). These wastepickers wait until the waste is collected and dumped at the site and then they scavenge through the waste for materials that can be recycled for money. Although the wastepicking may not be legal, cities allow the wastepickers to perform this task and even live on site. Ghana's Agbogbloshie is a large dump site for electronic waste. Wastepickers at that site collect the electronic material that has been dumped, such as laptops and cell phones, and harvest materials such as copper that can be found in cords and other metals and redeem these for money (Otsuka et al. 2012). Certainly the definition of wastepicker varies by country in terms of what is being collected and if these are formal or informal workers; but the fundamental concept of collecting materials that can be recycled and redeeming them for money is common around the world.

There are also various definitions of vulnerable populations, all of which apply to wastepickers. Vulnerable populations are a disadvantaged subgroup of society (Aday 1994). This is certainly true of wastepickers as they do not have the advantages of the formal labor market and they are from low socioeconomic conditions which in and of itself is a vulnerability. Many wastepickers have few years of education, which prevents them from entering the workforce or obtaining jobs with higher skill levels. While wastepicking provides an income, it often does not include employment benefits, and in some cases the recycling industry may take advantage of wastepickers (Auler et al. 2014). Likewise, wastepickers bear the risk of inclement weather, harassment from authorities and other citizens, and potential injuries from scavenging. A study of Nigerian wastepickers found that wastepickers were susceptible to injury and disease from rodents and insects that lived in poorly stored waste (Afon 2007). Broken glass and other potentially harmful materials also pose a threat to wastepickers sorting through trash to find redeemable cans or bottles. Adverse weather conditions, disease, and injury may also hinder or prevent a wastepicker from collecting bottles or cans. Since a wastepicker's income depends on his or her ability to collect recyclable waste, these occupational vulnerabilities threaten a wastepicker's livelihood.

Wastepickers have few resources to mitigate these risks. By not participating in the formal labor market they do not enjoy the protections afforded by labor laws, and may not have all the information needed to make informed choices. These vulnerabilities can be exacerbated if wastepickers live in informal housing, lack sanitation systems, or experience food insecurity. Vulnerabilities are also increased if wastepickers are immigrants, particularly those without legal permission to be in a country, as they are performing a valuable service for that society but have limited legal protection in the society. Fear of deportation also adds to vulnerability. All these factors make wastepickers an economically and socially vulnerable subgroup in a society (Auler et al. 2014). Vulnerable groups need special attention if their situation is to be improved, meaning their needs must be understood and their challenges should demand solutions. More importantly, vulnerable groups like wastepickers deliver a useful service and there needs to be a recognition of their contribution to society. In order to gain an understanding of the multi-dimensionality of the lives of groups like wastepickers, we need to comprehend the different facets of their lives and livelihood from their point of view. In doing so, we also need to be mindful of ethical considerations regarding research with vulnerable groups.

Motivation Our study team wanted to learn about the health of wastepickers in the United States. This group is of particular interest due to their vulnerability, the existence of laws for redeeming recycling which provides income, and even though this group has rarely been studied they are important in the economic and environmental services they provide. New York is one of the states that has a redemption law otherwise known as the Bottle Bill (Levitt and Leventhal 1986). A five cent deposit is included in the price of most beverage containers sold to final consumers by a retailer. Consumers or anyone with an empty beverage container may return the empty container to retailers, redemption machines, or redemption centers and get back the five cents. Although there are a variety of redemption centers in New York City, only one is a non-profit. This non-profit redemption center, called Sure We Can (SWC), is committed to community improvements in Brooklyn and environmental sustainability. As a result, this center provides an excellent opportunity to study the health of wastepickers, locally called canners, using a community based participatory framework.

Community-based participatory research (CBPR) is an approach to research that is grounded in collaborative equitable partnerships through the entire research process (Minkler and Wallerstein 2011). It is an asset-based approach to research (Green and Haines 2015) which recognizes and acknowledges the resources and strengths available in a community and leverages these assets for positive change. Since it is change oriented, CBPR seeks to balance research needs with positive action for its partners. Furthermore, we conceived and implemented this CBPR project with an interdisciplinary group of researchers which allowed us to holistically consider the issue of health and healthcare utilization of canners in NYC.

6.2 Process

The participatory process followed by Pennsylvania State University (PSU) researchers and SWC unfolded over several months in 2016 and 2017. On our first visit to SWC in March 2016, we met with Ana De Luco, one of the co-founders of Sure We Can, the only non-profit can redemption center in the New York City area. The PSU researchers wanted to connect with SWC and express interest in working with canners in New York City. Fortunately, Ana was interested in exploring how we could develop a project to examine the health utilization of canners of SWC. Ana was motivated because, even though SWC had partnered with several higher education institutions and nonprofits, they did not at that moment have any initiatives focused on health. She was looking for opportunities to find out more about the health care needs of the canners that used the services of SWC and she hoped that our project would fulfill this need. Thus, began our interdisciplinary collaboration with SWC. In addition to having an interdisciplinary group of researchers from PSU partnering with SWC, we involved graduate and undergraduate students in several stages of the project.

This underscores the fact, that for any fruitful participatory process, all parties require their needs to be satisfied. The PSU researchers wanted to understand the health status and the healthcare needs of canners in NYC, while SWC wanted to find out more about the health needs of its community so that they could provide better services to the canners that used their facility. The PSU researchers also wanted to use this project to offer research opportunities to Penn State students and expose them to community based research.

Community Partner: Sure We Can
- SWC is a non-profit recycling center, community space and sustainability hub in Brooklyn, New York where canners, who are people that collect cans and bottles from streets to make a living, come together with students and neighbors through recycling, composting, gardening and arts.
- Their mission is to support the local community, particularly the most vulnerable residents, and promote social inclusion, environmental awareness and economic empowerment. For over 9 years, Sure We Can has served the community of canners, and today it has evolved into a community center that promotes a sustainable urban culture and facilitates a circular economy.
- More than 500 canners are part of their community, collecting over ten million cans and bottles last year (2016) alone.

The majority of the wastepickers in our proposed study population were immigrants. Migration, and the health of migrants, are an important component of global health. As we described our study to our PINGH colleagues we learned about our partners who had worked with informal workers. We wanted to learn from our partners in Pune, India at the Savitribai Phule Pune University (SPPU), who have a long-standing relationship with a wastepicker organization in the city (Kagad Kach Patra Kashtakari Panchayat – KKPKP). The wastepickers in Pune are organized, have a long history and work with the municipality to collect and process household waste. Even though the Pune waste pickers collect a wider range of products we wanted to learn from the experience of an organized group of waste-pickers. However, the timing of activities between the PSU team and the SPPU team and the geographical distance proved to be very challenging. We were unable to complete a multi-sited project between the two groups, but will leverage our findings and lessons from the US to develop the next phases of research targeting both sites. We plan to collect additional data in India and Ghana, through PINGH partners.

Collaborative and equitable partnership From the onset, SWC stressed that this project needed to be a collaborative partnership. Since Ana was in the process of handing over the reins of SWC to Agustina Besada – who was taking over as the Executive Director of SWC – Ana introduced us to Agustina who then served as the main contact for SWC for the project. We first met with Agustina in August 2016, and between August 2016 and March 2017 – the PSU research team met with Agustina and SWC representatives regularly to establish a working relationship and to develop the research process/protocol for the study. This collaborative process was crucial for the development of trust between the research team and SWC. It also led to the development of a feasible study protocol that would be useful for all involved partners. Agustina was involved in all stages of the research process. We had several discussions regarding the research questions driving the study and the methodology to be followed. We collectively made decisions regarding questions to include in the survey and semi-structured questionnaire and the particulars of the methods to be used. For example, initially, the research team was interested in piloting the use of GPS devices to understand the routes taken by individual canners. However, Agustina was not sure of using GPS trackers and thought that some canners would be distrustful of such a method and it might compromise the entire research study. So ultimately, instead of using GPS trackers, we decided to use a map of the SWC neighborhood to solicit information about their canning route. Canners described the route that they took most frequently and any important landmarks along this path.

Mutually helpful process Even though the research team's main interest was in understanding the healthcare status of canners, how they accessed health care services, and what could be done to improve healthcare utilization of this vulnerable group; the research protocol included questions that were of importance to SWC. The survey included a section on the experience that the canners had with Sure We Can services. The results of this section of the survey will assist SWC in improving the services that they provide to the canning community. Similarly, the

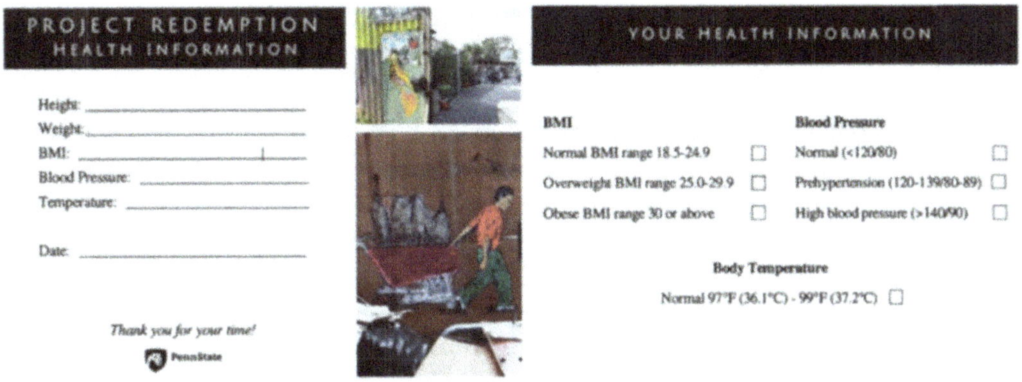

Fig. 6.1 Health information card with basic biometric measures was filled out and given to each participant taking part in the survey (front and back)

qualitative interview included questions about SWC and how the organization helped them and could improve the services that they provided to the canners. We were also committed to provide the study participants with something of utility – so that they would gain something immediately from the project beyond helping us understand their healthcare status and healthcare utilization patterns. After the survey we provided the participants with some basic information regarding their health status in the form of a health card that we handed back to them (see Fig. 6.1). Participants could use this to self-monitor any conditions, or use it as a reference point when visiting a health provider.

Asset-based Approach In developing the questions for the survey and the qualitative interviews, we were careful to not focus solely on deficiencies or unmet needs of the canners (Green and Haines 2015). Accordingly, the survey probed into the different dimensions of canning, including how the activity of canning and SWC positively impacted their lives. In the same vein, the qualitative questions asked the canners about the benefits of canning to the individual canners as well as the community. This was predicated on the belief that canning is a sustainable, useful income-generating activity and not necessarily an act of last resort. This was corroborated by the individual stories of canners: for example, one of the canners picked up cans for fun and exercise. He had a regular job, but engaged in canning for an hour or two every day to give him an excuse to walk around the city and to talk to people who he would otherwise not talk to in the process of his daily activities.

Interdisciplinary Approach This study was shaped from the very beginning by an interdisciplinary approach. The PSU researchers represented various disciplinary (and professional) backgrounds: medical anthropology, health economics, and urban planning. Consequently, the study was conceptualized holistically – we wanted to look at canning as a productive activity that was both sustainable and at the same time linked to possible health hazards and exploitation. This also had implication for the research questions driving the study and the methodology used. The urban planner was interested in the spatial aspects of the canners lives – the routes that they took, and how the routes were related to their health utilization behavior. The anthropologist was keen to collect the stories of the canners – in their own voices, while the health economist wanted to find out about the health status of canners at SWC and the different dimensions of health care access and utilization. Accordingly, we used a mixed methods approach blending surveys with qualitative interviews that included mapping.

6.3 Challenges and Lessons Learned

The outcome of this extended collaboration building and data collection was a small but well-rounded mixed methods pilot study. We were able to identify key health issues and barriers among canners using the facilities at SWC. With the research team, students conducted brief health assessments, surveys, and qualitative interviews with 15 canners at Sure We Can.

One practice that we built into the process was the inclusion of students into all phases of research. Students seeking research experience assisted with the IRB submission, survey and qualitative interview design, data collection, and data analysis. One undergraduate student served as the research assistant (RA) for the project and was involved in all phases of the project. All of the students doing data collection had language skills to match the population of SWC canners, including English, Spanish, Mandarin, and Cantonese. They went through a half day training process on qualitative interviewing, conducted by professionals from the Center for Health Care and Policy Research at Pennsylvania State University. Rather than act as translators, students were able to speak directly with canners and remove a potential barrier to communication, while gaining valuable skills and experience. Further, a graduate student in Health Policy and Administration analyzed the study data to complete her master's thesis.

For the student RA, this was the first project in which she had the opportunity to engage in all aspects of research: from developing the research questions, getting IRB approval, recruitment, training, fieldwork/data collection, data analysis and writing. Her other research experiences involved working on data analysis and lab work, so this project served as her introduction to community based participatory research. She enjoyed this experience, and is looking to combine community-based research with her interest in photography and filmmaking as she thinks of her career path. When asked to comment on what had perhaps not worked so well and needed to be approached differently, she mentioned that she would have enjoyed a more active mentorship model, especially since as an undergraduate student this was a novel experience for her. This is a reminder for faculty to make time for their students and think intentionally of their role as mentors responsible for training the next generation of research practitioners. Another point the RA made was the need for more training in the methods of research in a cross-cultural context. Even though we trained students in undertaking survey and interview research under a community based research framework, we could have done a better job in developing cross-cultural competency. This would have probably helped the students in their interview/survey process and eased some of their anxiety. This is also a reminder of the sophistication of undergraduate student researchers and points to the need for faculty to involve undergraduate students in community based research practices, especially as it may shape their career trajectories. In a similar fashion, another undergraduate student characterized this experience as "unlike any other experience in college". He enjoyed the opportunity to work alongside a community (canners) about which relatively little is known.

The iterative and longitudinal process of developing a community partnership between faculty at PSU and colleagues at SWC has created a strong foundation. Our initial data collection has highlighted potential points of intervention and further study with canners, while solidifying the partners' desire to continue working together. We plan to replicate some parts of our study in other sites, while maintaining flexibility to understand informal workers in diverse contexts. Of particular note has been the successful inclusion of students across phases of the research process and emphasis on community assets. This model can assist others in developing community partnerships and working with vulnerable populations.

Challenges
- We faced challenges coordinating data collection across sites, and focused on one area for a pilot study.
- Truly engaged methodology is challenging with a vulnerable research population, due to language and accessibility.

Lessons Learned
- Using a nonprofit partner helps with managing issues of access, engagement, and relevance of research.
- Student involvement at all stages of the research process helps with training future researchers and minimizing the barriers of using translators during interviews.

Acknowledgements The authors thank the canners in the study, first and foremost, for sharing their time and experience with us. We also thank Sure We Can for their partnership, accommodation, and the important work they are doing. Additionally, the following Pennsylvania State University students were invaluable to the research process: Sarah Kidder, Tiange Chen, Tim Groh, Julian Orozco, Jingnan Miso, and Tianzhou Shen.

References

Aday LA (1994) Health status of vulnerable populations. Annu Rev Public Health 15(1):487–509. https://doi.org/10.1146/annurev.pu.15.050194.002415

Afon AO (2007) Informal sector initiative in the primary sub-system of urban solid waste management in Lagos, Nigeria. Habitat Int 31(2):193–204. doi.org/10.1016/j.habitatint.2007.02.007

Auler F, Nakashima ATA, Cuman RKN (2014) Health conditions of recyclable waste pickers. J Community Health 39:17–22. doi.org/10.1007/s10900-013-9734-5

BottleBill.org (2015) Bottle Bills in the USA: All US Bottle Bills. http://www.bottlebill.org/legislation/usa/allstates.htm. Accessed 25 Oct 2017

BottleBill.org (2016) Bottle Bills in the USA: New York. http://www.bottlebill.org/legislation/usa/newyork.htm. Accessed 25 Oct 2017

Chikarmane P, Narayan L (2000) Formalising livelihood: case of wastepickers in Pune. Econ Polit Wkly 35(41):3639–3642

Fiske CH (1983) The return to returnables: New York enacts a bottle bill. Pace Law Rev 4:141–167

Green GP, Haines A (2015) Asset building & community development. Sage Publications, Los Angeles

Hartmann CD (2013) Garbage, health, and well-being in Managua. NACLA Rep Am 46(4):62–65

Levitt L, Leventhal G (1986) Litter reduction: how effective is the New York State bottle bill? Environ Behav 18(4):467–479. doi.org/10.1177/0013916586184003

Medina M (2008) The informal recycling sector in developing countries: organizing waste pickers to enhance their impact. Gridlines; No. 44. World Bank, Washington, DC. https://openknowledge.worldbank.org/handle/10986/10586

Minkler M, Wallerstein N (eds) (2011) Community-based participatory research for health: from process to outcomes. Wiley, Hoboken

Otsuka M, Itai T, Asante KA et al (2012) Trace element contamination around the e-waste recycling site at Agbogbloshie, Accra City, Ghana. Interdiscip Stud Environ Chem Environ Pollut Ecotoxicol 6(6):161–167

Sarmiento H, Tilly C, de la Garza Toledo E, Gayosso Ramirez JL (2016) The unexpected power of informal workers in the public square: a comparison of Mexican and US organizing models. Int Labor Work Class Hist 89:131–152. doi.org/10.1017/S0147547915000368

Scheinberg A, Anschtz J (2006) Slim pickin's: supporting waste pickers in the ecological modernization of urban waste management systems. IJTMSD 5(3):257–270. doi.org/10.1386/ijtm.5.3.257/1

Chapter 7
Assessing Urban Health Data: A Case Study of Maternal and Child Health Data in Cape Town, South Africa

Caprice Knapp, Rebekka Mumm, Linda Skaal, and Ursula Wittwer-Backofen

7.1 Introduction

All over the globe, urbanization is occurring as towns become cities and cities become megacities. Megacities are cities that have 10 million or more inhabitants (United Nations 2014). As of 2017, there are 37 megacities in the world (New Geography 2017). It is estimated that by 2025, 66% of the world's population will live in cities (UN 2014). A substantial portion of that growth, or 37%, is anticipated to come primarily from cities in India, China, and Nigeria (UN 2014). As urbanization persists, public and private organizations, as well as citizens, must grapple with the impacts and prepare for the future.

Although each city has its unique structure and dynamic, they all face the situation of areas of high population densities within city borders. Health services are often inaccessible for the urban poor due to a lack of financial resources and information, long distances to health services, or cultural and linguistic incompatibility. As a result, the urban poor can experience health and health system disparities (WHO 2010). Coordinating efforts to improve the health of the urban poor requires a detailed knowledge of the health needs of the urban poor in specific geographic areas of a city and comparing those needs to existing resources to identify gaps. Comprehensive information, including local-level data, is needed to improve the

C. Knapp (✉)
Department of Health Policy and Administration, Pennsylvania State University, State College, PA, USA
e-mail: ck47@psu.edu

R. Mumm · U. Wittwer-Backofen
Faculty of Medicine, Biological Anthropology, Center for Medicine and Society, University of Freiburg, Freiburg im Breisgau, Germany

L. Skaal
Department of Public Health, University of Limpopo, Polokwane, South Africa

© The Author(s) 2018
M. S. Winchester et al. (eds.), *Global Health Collaboration*, SpringerBriefs in Public Health, https://doi.org/10.1007/978-3-319-77685-9_7

health of people living in urban areas. We explored the possibilities for obtaining urban health data in South Africa, focusing on maternal and child health, embedded within context. Similar to the layers of the ecological model, comprehensive urban health data requires information across multiple levels.

A number of international and national organizations promote the principles of healthy cities. Goal 11 of the United Nation's (UN) Sustainable Development Goals is to, "make cities inclusive, safe, resilient, and sustainable" (UN 2017). The goal has targets for housing, transport systems, inclusive participation, cultural and natural heritage, deaths caused by disasters, adverse environmental impact, green and public spaces, regional development planning, integrated policies and plans, and sustainable and resilient buildings. The World Health Organization (WHO) supports health and sustainable development in cities by not only focusing on the health and health care infrastructure in cities, but also on the contribution of health care facilities on waste, pollution, and energy consumption (WHO 2017). WHO, UN, and other organizations have available resources for the promotion of healthy cities and for facilitation of actors in urban health related decision-making.

Understanding the complex intersections of urbanization and health is therefore a major requirement for successful approaches to improve urban health. A comprehensive conceptual framework can help to orient academics, researchers, and health policy makers to the same page and a common language. Among various existing models, we follow Bronfenbrenner and Morris' (2006) conceptual model to explain the factors that affect urban health. Similar to other bioecological approaches, their model shows that health for an individual or a group is impacted by the following broad levels: individual, social and community networks, environment, and society.

Mothers and their children are a specific group that can be studied using this conceptual model. Maternal and child health is a major area of interest for health, medicine, and public health for international and national organizations, as well as non-governmental and governmental organizations. Maternal health is concerned with outcomes such as maternal mortality, birth and pregnancy-related outcomes, perinatal mental health, feeding choices, or teenage pregnancies. Child health concerns issues such as infant and child mortality, nutrition, growth and development, early childhood disease, and immunization.

In order to apply the model, individual factors such as age, gender, and race or ethnicity, need to be included. Social and community factors include family support systems and health facilities that are nearby. Environment factors include where a person lives, works, and engages in recreational activity. Societal factors include culture, socioeconomic, and government. The model shows that these levels are linked, and that they have mediating and/or moderating effects on health.

7.1.1 Data

Urban health data use, otherwise known as health informatics, is the intersection of information science and urban health. The three building blocks of informatics are: data, information, and knowledge. In the urban health context, these building blocks and the interplay between them, can be quite complex. First, data must be generated and captured. Referring back to Bronfenbrenner's model it is clear that data from each of the factors is distinct. Environmental health data that describe the amount of indoor particulates is generated in a distinctly separate manner than spatial data on the amount of green space in a city. Each of the Bronfenbrenner factors has distinct data types that are generated and captured in a unique manner and by a variety of organizations. Issues that arise in the data are related to structure, standardization, accuracy, variability, integration, coordination, and costs of collection and processing.

An example of the need for integrated and coordinated data can be seen in monitoring the health of people living in urban areas. Suppose that a city wants to monitor the number of children who are not meeting basic standards for growth and development. It could be the case that one area of the city, perhaps a district within the city, has this data readily available and ready to use. However, this would only represent a small sample of the cities' children. In the absence of a mandate or widespread guidelines, districts might have collected the growth and development data based on different definitions, applying different methods for data sampling and handling, or otherwise. This would make it extremely difficult for the city to get a clear picture of the situation. One solution would be policies that allow for the integrated and coordinated management of growth and development data across the city. Although this seems straightforward, it can be costly, complex, and must compete with other health care priorities such as care delivery.

Once the data is collected, it needs to be converted to information. Again, for each of the Bronfenbrenner factors this is distinct. Public and private organizations direct the conversion of data to information based on their priorities. For example, the WHO publishes a Mental Health Atlas (WHO 2015b) that describes services available by country. Most of the conversion from data to information happens within the agency that collected the data as a way to address their own priorities. Issues on converting data to information are related to accuracy, availability, bias, access, adequacy, usability, transferability, dissemination, and costs related to processing.

The conversion of information to knowledge and further to an intervention in order to improve the situation is the final step and the ultimate goal. Data and information are used to gain knowledge and this knowledge results in advancement of urban health. In a public health approach, usually a cascade of steps is followed in a logical order to reach the goal (see Table 7.1). This is often demonstrated by testing interventions, or a variety of interventions about the same topic, over time. With each test, information is gained and overall this results in knowledge. An example from urban health is maternal mortality among poor urban women. Suppose one inner city hospital collects birth vital statistics for each birth (this is data). A researcher may notice poor women seem to have worse outcomes than those who are not poor. This can be investigated by comparing descriptive information of the average maternal mortality for poor versus non-poor women in the hospital for the past 5 years (this is information). Finding evidence that poor women have higher maternal mortality, the researcher tests whether having a midwife lowers maternal mortality. Assuming that the midwife intervention indicates that the result is positive, meaning maternal mortality is lower with a midwife (this is knowledge). The issues related to knowledge

Table 7.1 Public Health steps in the conversion of information to knowledge combining Public Health models based on Gibney et al. 2004 and Kroeger et al. 2004, adapted to a maternal health setting: From Information to an increase in Knowledge in Public Maternal Health

Step	Action		Example case study
1	Collect data		Hospital collects vital statistics for each birth
2	Identify health related problem		Compare maternal mortality between poor and non-poor city districts
3	Set goal		Reduce maternal mortality to one half in 10 years
4	Define objectives for goal		Achieve this reduction in mortality by midwife intervention
5	Create quantitative targets		Provide pregnant women with at least two antenatal health care and birth interventions by midwifes
6	Develop program		Develop a net of community health units and promotion materials
7	Implement program		Send out health worker to inform families
8	Evaluate program		Recording maternal mortality, add a risk factor analysis by using demographic and socioeconomic data, analyse and discuss

are about how interventions can be tested, how to pool results from a number of interventions, dissemination, reproducibility, generalizability, and costs.

Of course, there is more to urban health data than these three building blocks Data-Information-Knowledge, for which the term of health informatics might apply better. Informatics is additionally concerned with the systems used to generate and capture the data. Systems are typically clinical, administrative, and public health. Clinical systems include electronic health records and pharmacy management, administrative include billing and human resources, and public health includes surveillance. Workforce is also important in informatics whereby there should be adequate numbers with appropriate skills. Programmers, developers, data analysers, and quality improvement managers are examples of jobs that are needed in urban health informatics. Finally, informatics is concerned with privacy, security, and governance. At the individual level, privacy is always a concern when dealing with health data. Citizens want to be sure that their data is used in a way that has the least risk for loss of confidentiality and that the minimal amount of information necessary is shared. Organizations must take steps to guard their data and this has become more important recently facing worldwide hacking attacks. In many countries national, state, and local laws exist that are specifically directed at health care organizations with the intent to protect personal and sensitive health data. Ethical review boards also seek to ensure that researchers protect the privacy of participant data and their confidentiality. As informatics creates data, and then converts that data to information and knowledge, issues of privacy and security are of the upmost importance.

Governance refers to the chain of ownership of data and its accessibility. This is an area in urban health informatics that is rarely addressed, but is critical. For example, data on traffic related deaths might be collected by the Department of Motor Vehicles. However, if this data is needed for an urban health research project then it needs to be accessible. This is often difficult in that agencies are protective of their data, limit use of their data, and often do not make it publicly available. Even when data can be accessed, the urban health researcher must have a comprehensive data dictionary, particularly if the data come from a field that is unfamiliar. Governance also comes into concern when researchers want to match datasets. Suppose that two data sets are available at the individual level, it would be optimal to match those datasets but identifying information is needed. Matches made on name, birthdate, and address alone are not as accurate as those are where a unique identifier is also included. However, in countries where there is a large number of informal workers, personal identifiers might not be used in a high enough frequency or even available. More common is the case where researchers want to match data on a geographic level. For example, if a researcher wants to describe an outbreak of malaria in an urban poor area it might be good to do so by neighbourhoods or a unit smaller than district. This can be difficult as available data, and even the manner in which data are collected and processed, might not be accessible at the neighbourhood level. In general, the smaller the available units the more useful the data are for urban health.

7.2   Urban Maternal and Child Health as a Focus

Evolutionary aspects play an important role in changing environments such as urban challenges are. Adaptation to environments via genetic selection processes, leading to an adaptive increase in population frequencies of those genes who provide the carrier with beneficial traits, help to guarantee survival in the long run. Whereas the development of genetic and behavioural coping strategies are crucial for an optimal environmental embedding, evolutionary adaptation trends are often slow adaptive procedures over many generations, and do not contribute to an understanding of how urban populations are able to cope with the fast-changing urban environments. Throughout human history, highest rates of vulnerability in a population were reached under changing environments (such as the transition from foraging to sedentary life, the formation of medieval cities, or the early industrialization), when the evolved coping capacities did not fit to the environmental challenges any more, which nowadays is the case in urban environments permanently (Nonini 2014). Short term adaptations as studied only recently with the field of epigenetics reacting to environmental conditions suggest that fast and meaningful reactions occur affecting the activity of genes. As these activation patterns seem to inherit to the next generation, the influence of environmental factors might be even much more effective than it has been assumed until recently.

This is especially evident if considering meaningful behavior of mothers significantly affecting their offspring. First studies e.g. suggest an epigenetic influence on the relationship between urban upbringing and social stress processing fixed by neural regulation in the brain (Lederbogen et al. 2011).

Besides others, these first results suggest that the environmental influence on mothers and their children is even higher than expected compared to the classical risk factors models. This is a clear demand to care for mother and child health in urban environments, suggesting to invest much of our global health capacities into mother and child population subgroups.

Focusing on urban maternal and child health adds on the complexities of living in an urban environment. A variety of factors could affect health of mothers and children such as social determinants of health, health systems, environment, community, social networks, etc. Often maternal and child urban studies focus on vulnerable populations including migrants, poor, disabled, single mothers, and those with mental health conditions. Regardless of whether maternal and child health is viewed for an entire urban population or specific subgroups are targeted, it is an important investment for governments and other key stakeholders in communities, because maternal & child mortality is an indication of a country's health systems failure or success (UNICEF 2016).

For many years, academics, governments, and non-governmental organizations have investigated different programs, policies, and interventions to improve maternal and child health. As a result, much progress has been made in most developed countries compared to under-developed countries. The U.S. Agency of International Development (USAID) notes that since 2008 their 24-country partnership with the WHO has saved the lives of 4.6 million children and 200,000 women (USAID 2016). Polio has been eradicated from India through a number of surveillance and vaccination efforts (Obregon et al. 2009). The United Nations' Millennium Development Goal led to a reduction in under-five mortality from 12.7 million to 6 million between 1990 and 2015 and the maternal mortality rate has fallen by 44 per cent (WHO 2015b). These are just some examples out of many that have contributed to making the lives of mothers and children better. Commitment of governments to ensure sustained progress in reducing under-five mortality and the maternal mortality rates and bridging the existing access to health care disparities is but one the crucial methods of sustaining healthy communities.

The heart of this progress is data, information, and knowledge. Without these three pillars it would be impossible to track, monitor, and evaluate any progress in maternal and child health. It would also be difficult to understand where and how to intervene and how to formulate effective policies and encourage effective practices. Advancing maternal and child health requires data, yet data collection is expensive and often done in a haphazard manner. Data collection is typically done to answer a targeted question without regard for how new disciplines could utilize the data in the future. Finally, data collection is moot unless those data are ultimately turned into information and knowledge. Data should be and bring about concrete change.

For urban maternal and child health, the most optimal scenario would be that organizations would collect data in an informed, interdisciplinary manner and be able to demonstrate the conversion into information and knowledge, which leads to improved outcomes. Certainly, reality is often different from the best-case scenario. The following case study describes an attempt to assess the maternal and child data in South Africa.

7.3 Maternal and Child Health in South Africa

7.3.1 Setting

Considerable investments have been made in maternal and child health data management in South Africa. South Africa has governmental, academic, and community infrastructure facilities that are active in maternal and child health suggesting that this country would be able to source and monitor data on child and maternal health. Despite advancements in maternal and child health, South Africa still has significant numbers of under-five mortality or mother-child HIV transmission (Groenewald et al. 2014; Cock et al. 2000) so the interest to improve data capturing and management persists.

Disparities in access to health have been in existence pre- and post-apartheid in this country, which unfortunately impact directly on the quality of health data that exist, and on the dissemination and translation to practice. For example, national data on child and maternal health do not include data from private sectors, making it impossible to accurately report on the status of the country with regard to this (Weimann et al. 2016). According to a study by Oni and Mayosi (2016), gaps in data management on the subject exist, at province and even at country level, underreporting on both child and maternal mortality rates.

In Limpopo, a rural province in SA, public hospitals do not properly report maternal mortality, because there are no standardised tools to accurately document maternal mortality. Additionally, some pregnant patients are admitted in different wards (not maternity wards) for other ailments, and when they die in those wards, they are not recorded as maternal mortality cases. In those tertiary hospitals where mortality recording tools are in place, there is a paucity of information that is recorded, depending on the experience of the person who is recording the incidence of maternal mortality.

There is an urgent need to focus on *urban* health in South Africa as four of the top 20 fastest growing cities in Africa are located in South Africa such as Cape Town (African Development Bank Group 2014). At the heart of this growth, migration to this city has been increasing in large proportions, in a quest to seek employment opportunities.

Therefore, our health data analysis reflects the current conditions within a specific urban setting and does not allow a conclusion concerning other African settings. We rather emphasize the value of health relevant data and identify existing data and their structure, as well as recognizing data gaps.

Finally, this in-depth analysis of maternal and child urban health data was part of a larger study which was focused on Cape Town. The aim of the study was a health gap analysis as a contribution to understand the health situation and to explore, to which health issues attention is paid to, what neglected diseases occur, or what neglected health issues are missing in the focus of researchers (Mumm et al. 2017). Thus, such a health gap analysis allows an overview over existing information and data and represents a mirror of the capacity of the health system. Among the major results the gap analysis revealed a clear gap in the field of maternal mental health in the city of Cape Town, a much-needed health service as a clear sign of unfavourable living conditions for mothers and their children. As well the intercultural approach allows a view on a regional setting with a different perspective as approached by the local authorities and health workers.

7.3.2 Methods and Aims

Two approaches were used to assess the maternal and child urban health data in South Africa: a literature review and the identification, cataloguing, and statistical analyses of available datasets. Identification and cataloguing of datasets help to understand what data are available and the characteristics of that data. The project was primarily focused on secondary datasets that exist and are known publicly. This also speaks to the transparency of data in the country. Many other urban health datasets exist but one objective of the project was to demonstrate what can be explored with the available data and used by a larger audience that seeks to understand, study, and improve the situation. The literature review aims to understand how data has been converted into information and knowledge. A major objective of studying these two columns of information was to see if the situation analysis based on each of the information columns delivers the same picture or a different picture of the urban maternal and child health situation in Cape Town.

7.3.3 Literature Review

In order to summarize the available mother-child health datasets in South Africa a narrative review of the literature was conducted in May 2015. Child health growth indicators were also catalogued from the literature review. PubMed, Google Scholar, National Center for Biotechnology Information (NCBI) were used to search online for relevant literature in the fields of anthropology and health including the sub-disciplines of public health and global health. Further reviews were done on the homepage of journals that were applicable to the topic.

Because structured search terms were used, additional literature in "other" fields beyond the ones listed above were also searched. Search terms were reviewed and agreed upon by the research team. These include: *children health, neonatal health, growth, obesity, overweight, infant mortality, weight-for-height, height-for-age, weight-for-age, BMI-for-age, stunting, wasting, infant development, maternal health, maternal, pregnancy, urban health, mother-child health, health care system, smoking during pregnancy, and foetal alcohol syndrome*. Boolean operators were used in the online searches to ensure that the results were applicable, for example "urban health + children health". Geographic search terms were also used including Cape Town, Western Cape, South Africa, Sub-Saharan Africa, and Africa. Although these terms include some broader (Africa) and narrower (Cape Town) geographic areas they were used to ensure that all applicable literature was reviewed. Titles, abstracts, and full papers were extracted and read according to Cochrane guidelines. All applicable literature was catalogued and, if raw data were mentioned and publicly available, attempts were made to gain access to the datasets. The following information was extracted for each publication to the database; title, year published, author(s), indicators, aggregation level, data source, sample size, location, availability, and contact details of author(s). Specific child growth data were extracted including; age and ethnicity of participants, growth measurements, and references to other studies.

7.3.4 Datasets

Based on the literature review several potential data sources were identified that were either suitable for a primary or secondary data analysis on mother and child health. Primary data analysis was done on accessible raw data provided by contacted persons. Due to a low response rate and the focus on analysing information gaps (secondary data analysis) solely raw data of the Western Cape Mortality Report (Groenewald et al. 2014) were analysed which include number of death per age, cause of death and geographic region. This dataset was used to calculate infant and under five mortality rates and mortality rates of women in childbearing ages. Information to calculate maternal mortality was missing due to missing data on causes of death.

Availability of secondary data was far higher and covers all the intended areas of interest from South Africa to the Western Cape region to Cape Town and even city districts within Cape Town. General information such as life expectation, sanitary, housing, age distribution were available from census data (Statistics South Africa 2011) provided by the South African Government. Access to raw data was not possible on all levels.

Although most of the datasets refer to mother-child health, information was diverse in density of details, studied population, content, and indicators used to describe mother-child health. In general, published articles or information either included information on maternal health (e.g. mortality rates, HIV and tuberculosis prevalence) or on child health (e.g. mortality and morbidity rates, growth, and vaccination). No studies were found that assessed the health of mother-child dyads in South Africa, independent on level of aggregation. However, this type of information is necessary to describe the risk factors and the vulnerability of mothers and children and to provide sufficient interventions to improve mother-child health. In addition, although mortality and morbidity were surveyed, they were not matched with data on living conditions, access to health care and other factors that might explain the observed prevalence for diseases and mortality rates. Without this combined information, intervention programs may not reach their potential as they may not be tailored for the needs of the community.

Furthermore, availability of datasets strongly depends on the level of aggregation. For example, the smaller the studied geographic aggregation, the less detailed information may be available. For Cape Town, its eight health districts were the smallest level on which at least some information could be accessed. Information for smaller communities with their special cultural and socioeconomic conditions within the city was not available. An overview of the available secondary data, in relation to aggregation level, is presented in Table 7.2.

Besides data availability and accessibility, the review also allowed for comments on data quality. As in other countries, published information from South Africa often does not include information on study design or data quality assurance making it difficult to be critically reviewed. For example, the maternal mortality rate in Cape Town is the highest in high-socioeconomic districts whereas it is the lowest in low-socioeconomic districts characterized by informal settlements, no clear drinking water and less access to health care. Without understanding the methodology for how the data was collected and analysed, or perhaps potential biases, the meaning of this finding might be misconstrued. A simple reason could be that high-socioeconomic districts have greater resources for reporting birth vital statistics than low-socioeconomic districts.

The crucial aspect for all countries is the ability to record accurate data for maternal and child health outcomes, from which interventions can be drawn. In most African countries, there is poverty of reliable data on the subject, as a result, in most cases data on both maternal and child health outcomes is undocumented or incompletely documented (Mumm et al. 2017). The fact that there is no suppository bank linking both public and private sector, makes it impossible for countries to accurately report the status of child and maternal health which is always marred by underreporting on maternal mortality.

7.4   Reflections

In order to understand what information is available concerning maternal and child health and how it can be used, an exercise was planned and conducted that focused on Cape Town and on a broader view on South Africa. However, any city could have been chosen with similar or more disparate results. South Africa was chosen because it was supposed to represents, most likely, the best case scenario of available data on the African continent (see above). However, the ever-changing impact of urbanization due to economic, political, and cultural changes needs to be constantly considered in the urban health subject.

Table 7.2 Available secondary data on mother and child health in South Africa (SA), in the province Western Cape (WC), in the city of Cape Town (CT), and in city health districts (CTHD) by aggregation level

Field of information	SA	WC	CT	CT HD
Demographic information				
Area	x	x	x	x
Population	x	x	x	x
Population density	x	x	x	x
Number & size of households	x	x	x	x
Life expectancy	x	x	x	x
Number & cause of deaths	x	x	x	x
Age distribution and ethnicities	x	x	x	x
Male-female ratio		x		x
Total fertility rate	x	x		
Age of mother at birth	x	x	x	
Mortality rates				
Infant mortality rate	x	x	x	x
Under-5 mortality rate	x	x	x	x
Maternal mortality rate	x	x	x	x
Socioeconomic information				
Average income	x			x
Education	x	x		x
Housing & sanitation	x			x
Food security	x			
Unemployment rate	x	x		x
(Maternal) Health care				
Availability (density) of health facilities	x	x	x	x
Access to health care	x			
Utilization of health care	x			
Prevalence of communicable & non-communicable diseases	x	x		(x)
Immunization of children	x	x		
Level of & access to perinatal care	x	(x)	(x)	
HIV prevalence – adults & children	x	x	x	
HIV prevalence – pregnant women & mothers	x			
Number of antiretroviral therapy – adults & mothers	x			
Nutritional status of children	x	x		
Health risks of adults – alcohol & tobacco	x	x		

Sources see Mumm et al. (2017)

x data fully available on aggregation level, (x) data incompletely available

Datasets and available literature were reviewed to understand the situation of mother-child health in South Africa. Particular attention was paid to what datasets were referred to, if they were available, and analyses were conducted on some of these available datasets. Based on the planning, execution, and reflection of the project, several lessons learned are listed below.

There was a plethora of data on urban mothers and children in South Africa and specifically in Cape Town. However, the data were often uncoordinated, not differentiated between situation analysis, and it was unclear if these data would be useful for meaningful development of strategies and implementation of health improvement programs. Across the different datasets that were available, there was often a mismatch in the data structure and aggregation levels. Differing definitions of terms prevented comparison across datasets and sometimes data was collected at only the national level and sometimes at more discrete geographic units. While national data can provide insights for stakeholders on what needs to be improved, finer level data are needed to understand where and how to start with targeted interventions.

Data availability impacts its usefulness and transparency. Although there are issues related to propriety around sharing data, the study team received no responses back from inquiries made about obtaining primary datasets that were cited in the literature review. Governments might require that datasets collected using public funds be available, at least in a limited manner, for use by the public. Use of data by the public, not just academics, is important for meaningful change. During the literature review it was clear that data, information, and knowledge on urban health for mothers and children are publicly available, but not easy to locate or in a number of unrelated sources such as journals, websites, or in grey publications. However, recently there has been a specialized focus on urban health journals, on maternal and child health, as well as on the health issues of Africa. Although the interest of the study was the intersection of all three areas, these specifically focused resources make information access easier. It was interesting to note that there was a lack of visibility of interdisciplinary research on urban health or the study of maternal and child health from a comprehensive perspective. It is possible that data are not being using in the most powerful way. Given that some data were not available at levels smaller than national, it would be difficult to use those to facilitate change in a smaller unit such as a city, community or district.

Since we followed the WHO definition of health as a state of complete physical, mental and social well-being and not merely the absence of disease or infirmity (WHO 1948), the search for data, information and knowledge on mother and child health in South Africa and specifically in Cape Town included a comprehensive approach. Although in many cases the aims of data collections were not clearly documented, we found the majority of approaches on physical health, assuming that this field received higher priorities compared to mental health. As the focus on mother and child health requires a comprehensive approach, a fruitful interaction of scientists from diverse disciplines, as it was the case in this project, is needed. The team of researchers met this challenge of developing a better culture of communication between humanities and Life Sciences/Medicine, or between different scientific cultures, including seeking for an integrative and balanced significance of both quantitative and qualitative approaches. Such skills in health approach interactions need to be actively developed, are often time-consuming, or suffer from a lack of suitable funding options. But this is the most promising approach of dealing with the highly complex and dynamic processes interacting in the health situation of people in urban environments.

In closing, the lessons learned were somewhat expected. All countries, regardless of economic status, have improvements that are needed in data collection, analysis, and interpretation. Globally, there is a need in better understanding and improving health in an evidence-based manner. Perhaps the lessons learned would have been different if the study had been conducted by in-country researchers only. However, given that data, information, and knowledge production are important around the world, the lessons learned can be applied in many different scenarios and are important for stakeholders to consider in planning and decision making.

Challenges
- Across the different datasets that were available, there was often a mismatch in the data structure and aggregation levels. Differing definitions of terms prevented comparison across datasets and sometimes data was collected at only the national level and sometimes at more discrete geographic units.
- While national data can provide insights for stakeholders on what needs to be improved, finer level data are needed to understand where and how to start with targeted interventions.

Lessons Learned
- As the focus on mother and child health requires a comprehensive approach, a fruitful interaction of scientists from diverse disciplines, as it was the case in this project, is needed.
- The team of researchers met this challenge of developing a better culture of communication between humanities and Life Sciences/Medicine, or between different scientific cultures, including seeking for an integrative and balanced significance of both quantitative and qualitative approaches.
- Such skills in health approach interactions need to be actively developed, are often time-consuming, or suffer from a lack of suitable funding options. But this is the most promising approach of dealing with the highly complex and dynamic processes interacting in the health situation of people in urban environments.

References

African Development Bank Group (2014) Tracking Africa's progress in figures. https://www.afdb.org/fileadmin/uploads/afdb/Documents/Publications/Tracking_Africa%E2%80%99s_Progress_in_Figures.pdf. Accessed 15 August 2017

Bronfenbrenner U, Morris P (2006) The bioecological model of human development. In: Lerner RM, Damon W (eds) Handbook of child psychology, Theoretical models of human development, vol 1, 6th edn. Wiley, New York

Cock KMD, Fowler MG, Mercier E et al (2000) Prevention of mother-to-child HIV transmission in resource-poor countries: translating research into policy and practice. JAMA 283(9):1175–1182. https://doi.org/10.1001/jama.283.9.1175

Gibney MJ, Margetts BM, Kearney JM, Arab L (eds) (2004) Public health nutrition. Blackwell Science, Oxford

Groenewald P, Msemburi W, Morden E et al (2014) Western Cape mortality profile. South African Medical Research Council, Cape Town, p 2011. http://www.mrc.ac.za/bod/WC2011Report.pdf. Accessed 11 October 2017

Kroeger A, Montoya-Aguilar C, Bichmann W et al (2004) The use of epidemiology in local health planning. A training manual. In: Zed Books. London, New Jersey

Lederbogen F, Kirsch P, Haddad L et al (2011) City living and urban upbringing affect neural social stress processing in humans. Nature 474(7352):498–501. https://doi.org/10.1038/nature10190

Mumm R, Diaz-Monsalve S, Hänselmann E et al (2017) Exploring urban health in Cape Town, South Africa: an interdisciplinary analysis of secondary data. Pathog Glob Health 111(1):7–22. doi.org/10.1080/20477724.2016.1275463

New Geography (2017) The 37 megacities and largest cities: demographia world urban areas: 2017. http://www.newgeography.com/content/005593-the-largest-cities-demographia-world-urban-areas-2017. Accessed 5 October 2017

Nonini DM (ed) (2014) A companion to urban anthropology. Wiley-Blackwell, Chichester

Obregón R, Chitnis K, Morry C et al (2009) Achieving polio eradication: A review of health communication evidence and lessons learned in India and Pakistan. Bull World Health Org 87(8):624–630. doi.org/10.1590/S0042-96862009000800020

Oni T, Mayosi BM (2016) Mortality trends in South Africa: progress in the shadow of HIV/AIDS and apartheid. Lancet Glob Health 4(9):e588–e589. doi.org/10.1016/S2214-109X(16)30178-4

Statistics South Africa (2011) Census 2011. http://www.statssa.gov.za/?page_id=993&id=city-of-cape-town-municipality. Accessed 15 August 2017

UN (2014) World urbanization prospects: the 2014 revision, highlights (ST/ESA/SER.A/352). https://esa.un.org/unpd/wup/publications/files/wup2014-highlights.Pdf. Accessed 15 August 2017

UN (2017) Sustinable Development Goals. https://www.un.org/sustainabledevelopment/

UNICEF (2016) Maternal and newborn health. https://www.unicef.org/health/index_maternal-health.html

USAID (2016) Shared progress, shared future. Agency financial report. https://www.usaid.gov/sites/default/files/documents/1868/USAIDFY2016_AFR_508.pdf. Accessed 6 October 2017

Weimann A, Dai D, Oni T (2016) A cross-sectional and spatial analysis of the prevalence of multi-morbidity and its association with socioeconomic disadvantage in South Africa: a comparison between 2008 and 2012. Soc Sci Med 163:144–156. doi.org/10.1016/j.socscimed.2016.06.055

WHO (1948) Preamble to the Constitution of WHO as adopted by the International Health Conference, New York

WHO (2010) Hidden cities: unmasking and overcoming health inequities in urban settings. http://www.who.int/kobe_centre/publications/hiddencities_media/who_un_habitat_hidden_cities_web.pdf. Accessed 2 May 2016

WHO (2015a) Mental health atlas, 2014. Department of Mental Health and Substance Abuse, World Health Organization, Geneva

WHO (2015b) Trends in maternal mortality: 1990 to 2015: estimates by WHO, UNICEF, UNFPA, World Bank Group and the United

WHO (2017). Safe management of wastes from health-care activities: a summary. World Health Organization. http://www.who.int/iris/handle/10665/259491

Chapter 8
Conclusion: Long Term Prospects and Global Health Collaboration

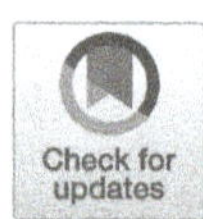

Nicole Webster

8.1 Introduction

The general direction of global health within academia seems to have moved to a stage where easily accessing information is vital to notions of transparency and interactions. The task of universities is to find and create pathways that inform society and our students about the realities of health across various nation states. While this might seem like a daunting task, the structure of Pan Institution Network for Global Health (PINGH) has provided avenues for exploring and addressing complex and interrelated health issues among global partners within an academic setting.

This book provides a platform for unpacking both the success and challenges faced by individuals in the academy (students, faculty, and administrators) and the communities in which they work in the world of global health. Published chapters reveal a collection and dissemination of performance, networks, systems, and people that contribute to the PINGH network and its goals. PINGH in its rawest form is a moving collection of parts and people working to achieve the goal of formalizing a network that enables local and national actors to address some of the world's most pressing health issues. In coordination with local agencies, hospitals, universities, and other key individuals, the network provides a type of methodology for engagement and problem-solving. In addition to hands-on engagement and experiences, the PINGH network serves as a space for nurturing and developing ideas. The network provides a domain for those who wish to test ideas or brings together like minds to address global health issues, while also creating pathways to the inclusion of diverse individuals, sectors of society, and communities in this complex and fast-paced field.

N. Webster (✉)
Department of Agricultural Economics, Sociology, and Education,
Pennsylvania State University, State College, PA, USA
e-mail: nsw10@psu.edu

© The Author(s) 2018
M. S. Winchester et al. (eds.), *Global Health Collaboration*, SpringerBriefs
in Public Health, https://doi.org/10.1007/978-3-319-77685-9_8

Another outcome of the chapters and primarily a result of the PINGH structure is an opportunity to advance the focus of global health collaborations and research with students and community partners. One might argue that this type of research already exists within other health-related organizations; however, the types of conversations, projects, and research carried out within PINGH highlight the impact that can happen when the community works with students in the co-creation of the knowledge and research. Take for example the Project Redemption project from Chap. 6, which highlights what can happen when communities that have often been overlooked are included as contributing participants and central to the core theme of the study. In other chapters (see Chaps. 4 or 7), the inclusion of undergraduate and graduate students was purposeful and impactful to not only the students but also provided useful information on potential changes that could ultimately influence how to better integrate students into other programmatic roles of these global health programs.

Furthermore, book chapters reveal challenges when working with global partners such as access and transparency of national data or access to other pertinent information. Despite these issues, authors recognized through these types of global health projects, greater awareness and policies (both PINGH and national/regional country policies) could be developed to address some of these limitations that impact programs. Another important issue raised across most chapters was the significance of a robust program design. When programs are strategically developed to include students (graduate and undergraduate), develop and challenge learning, incorporate community voice, and acknowledge critical reflection, there is an opportunity to change the status quo of student learning in global contexts. These components contribute to a learning environment that provides the student and the community with an opportunity to contribute to the learning process and ultimately create an experience that is meaningful to all.

In reviewing the system of PINGH and its goals, there were three common themes found in all the chapters. Projects and activities highlighted the elements of a network that values (1) community voice and inclusivity, (2) student engagement and contributions, and (3) faculty and site collaboration.

8.2 Community Voice and Inclusivity

Community participation in health care is vital and integral to the approaches and integration of the project. Community participation gives individuals a sense of being a part of the process and assisting in the development of research and or policies that will ultimately impact their health and livelihoods. As evidenced by the inclusion of the center director in the waste picker project or the community members in the diabetes research; the community was an integral part of the project, whether the authors noted successes or breakdowns in the process. What was consistent was the need to include the community as valued members of the process and not just program participants. Strategies to achieve healthy communities have viewed the inclusion of individuals such as community case managers or community health workers as critical components. The inclusion of the community in the case of these PINGH projects responded to community-level treatment and interventions for pressing issues that impact the community as a whole. As a result, activities focused on crucial essential elements necessary for including strategic community members (i.e. organizations, people, institutions), that would enable the implementation of the research or project. Attributes incorporated in PINGH projects which assisted in fostering community participation included the following:

- Contributing—community contributes time, expertise, and resources
- Consulting—community is asked for their views and knowledge
- Managing—community participates in making decisions and provides input

Although each PINGH project did not incorporate each of the three components mentioned above, they all displayed aspects of each element at specific points of time during the project. And while authors noted to hints of tension when working with the community, they expressed the desire and willingness in working with the community in a participatory manner.

Participatory and community processes are developed through the construction of trusting and collaborative relationships among all stakeholders, through inclusive actions. The relational work — sometimes mediating between different options or positions and in case of possible conflicts —is, therefore, a continuous and fundamental element. Construction and conduction of moments and meeting spaces and collaboration for the development of these initiatives, with the participation of citizens and technical-professional resources assisted in fostering program models that could be scaled up and replicated. Permanent listening and participatory research for a better and broader knowledge of the health conditions of the site areas led to more informed citizens and provided more significant information and socialization of community knowledge about health.

A review of the different interpretations of community participation shows a continuum that goes from the cooperative mode where the community provides information and manpower to more active and creative forms of participation in decision-making, negotiation, and presentation of proposals and co-administration of the resources. A vital aspect of these projects was the capacity and training built into the plans that facilitated participation by higher numbers of the community, leading to projects that have the potential for a sustainable future.

8.3 Student Engagement and Contributions

In the past decade, within higher education, there has been a growing conversation on the role and impact of students engaged in relevant and meaningful course content. Researchers have illustrated that student engagement is the most significant

Table 8.1 Engaged student learning

Meaningful and relevant program content	Students introduced to activities they believed as being useful and relevant to current academic program and future career goals
Fosters a sense of competence	Students are given opportunities to evaluate their personal growth and learning
Embraces collaborative learning	Activities enabled students to work with peers and community—Amplifying a sense of connection to others
Promotes mastery orientation or exposure	Student activities introduced them to new concepts/communities/activities or allowed them to develop further skills learned in classroom settings

predictor of retention and cognitive and personal development in college students (Belcheir 2000; Bridges et al. 2001; Nelson Laird et al. 2004; Kuh 2007). Studies also show that specific pedagogical practices are associated with higher levels of student engagement (Deakin Crick and Goldspink 2014). Student's engagement in society, their associations and networks, and the characteristics of their communities profoundly affect their outlook on life. The attributes commonly found in courses which engage youth in learning outside the classroom and in a global context incorporate some characteristics—structured participation; engagement with community organizations; connectedness with neighborhoods; and relationships with government and groups unlike one's own. Combined, they often contribute to positive learning outcomes and a deeper understanding of the systems and underlying history that adds to the health issues being studied.

Expanding this notion of engagement within the healthcare sector was most evident in many of the chapters. Authors discussed the multifaceted role of students in the projects, such as research associates, data organizers and collectors, and co-authors of research articles. In many cases, the students were engaging in work beyond what is typically carried out in engagement activities and even more so within the classroom. Students were exposed to research and projects that fostered conversations with organizations and community members who were able to provide context and meaning beyond a textbook. Moreover, students were assigned roles and responsibilities which could lead to personal growth and development.

In reviewing chapters which were intentional in the inclusion of students, both graduate, and undergraduates, each incorporated essential elements central to student engagement. Each project was mindful in the design and structure of the activity which led to students gaining greater knowledge of global health issues, exposure to various actors and determinants of health issues, and open dialogue and conversations with health professionals and others central to local and global advancements in global health. The intentionality in which each project approached the inclusion of students resulted in other components of engaged student learning (see Table 8.1).

Students' knowledge of the realities of global health was enhanced by their participation in the noted projects and further support the value of PINGH which provides support systems within colleges and units to foster this type of student learning.

8.4 Faculty and Site Collaboration: Fostering North-South Collaborations

Recognizing the value of understanding the interconnectedness and interactions of global health, the PINGH structure facilitates approaches for developing and fostering institutional relationships and collaborative research agendas. Although most projects were developed within the context of a PINGH meeting, they all expanded to reach out to global partners who may or may not have been at meetings. The goal is to create a project or research agenda that focused on an idea or universal health need. Conversations which formed the basis of these projects seemed to be done with the disposition of including multiple voices and perspectives. Participants and organizers approached their project with a sense of urgency and an understanding of their potential role in creating awareness of challenges that exist within areas of global health such as data collection methods, transparency of data, or improving the understanding in an evidence based material. Additional features of these projects leaned towards the role and importance of faculty in fostering global educational experiences for students, challenging the status quo of student learning beyond the traditional Western models of thinking and learning, and developing bilateral partnerships between students and emerging and experienced faculty.

The framework of PINGH enabled faculty and staff to consider conceptual frameworks that pressed learning environments to take place in both the Global North and South. Feasibility and specifications of learning sites and the relationship between these sites and selected social and global health trends aided in fostering these relations between countries. The inclusion of the north-south connection was not without challenges such as language barriers or understanding of cultural values and norms that impacted healthcare systems. But at the very least, participants were exposed to a different way of being and were able to co-construct knowledge with a diverse set of colleagues who held different sets of ideologies and systems.

The merit of these relationships was due to actions and behaviors that supported the engagement of individuals across and within various institutions and countries. Most notable were:

1. Conferences and workshops within multiple settings (US and abroad)

    (a) Discussion of ideas and potential projects took place in these settings
    (b) Training of emerging researchers and fostering support for all participants
    (c) Networking opportunities

2. Facilitation of small pilot grants to support projects/research

    (a) Enabled groups to continue noted work discussed at workshops/conferences

3. Transparent communication strategies

    (a) Newsletters, Skype calls

4. Interdisciplinary approach to project ideas

    (a) Several institutions part of a project

8.5   PINGH Network Structure and Recommendations

PINGH serves as a system which facilitates the fostering of ideas and advocates for activities related to global health. The success of the network clearly rests in the hands of all participants as well as the leadership. It is clear from the chapters that each project had a clear focus and goal that contributed to the success and helped to reveal potential areas of growth for PINGH members. As an organization designed to support multiple partners, it is clear that the structure encourages bilateral and multilateral programming to bring about informative and transformative changes to students, professionals, and most importantly to the global health community (see Fig. 8.1).

When examining the overarching structure and role of PINGH, it is an organization that can fill multiple gaps in the academia and the global health network. By providing educators, students, and the community with a framework, PINGH places value on the role of global health. A structure that supports ideas fosters collaboration and stimulates new avenues for existing, and emerging scholars situates the complexity of global health and the importance of cooperation and connectedness in addressing some of life's most challenging health issues. In light of this, what follow are a series of recommendations to continue to strengthen the existing partnerships of PINGH and develop more sustainable long term collaboration:

- For data collection and collaborative efforts with multiple partners, a multipronged strategy should be pursued in which large-scale surveys could be conducted by several institutions, providing greater opportunities for students, agencies, and the community at large. The greatest promise lies in research that has a longitudinal structure and includes avenues for exploring resources ranging from regional data to national data that are amenable to community-level analyses.
- Due to the importance of enhancing students' learning and advancement, greater avenues should be created to include students in the inclusion of projects to enhance both technical and leadership skills. Based on the projects that included students, there should be greater structures put in place to support their academic and research development further supporting them with experiences that have value beyond the classroom.
- The PINGH network should establish a technical team that assists the leadership team in further highlighting the global health research efforts. A technical team

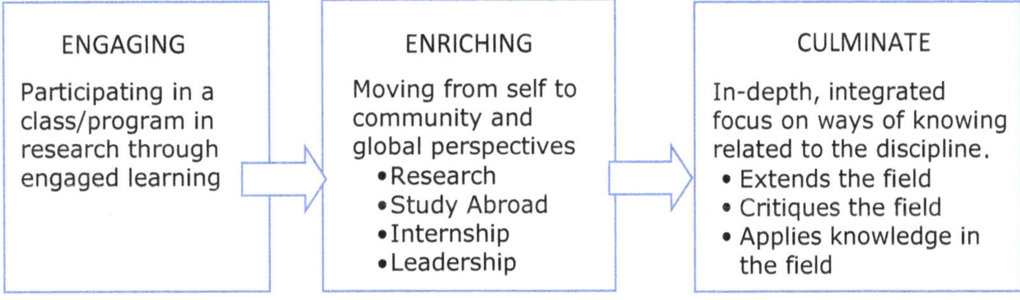

Fig. 8.1 PINGH network

could be led by graduate students, further fostering their social and technical skills and assisting them in building their networks of colleagues. This team could create strategies to promote research and other work being conducted through social media and other platforms to help develop a stronger tie between all the institutions.

– For fostering and monitoring relationships between emerging and seasoned researchers, an online platform could be developed to support these relationships. This component could assist in creating a system where content and resources are shared, and more importantly, housed for future reference. The platform may be especially helpful in moving forward creative and innovative ideas about types of research and opportunities that offer the most promise.

– In mapping the way forward for growing and managing partners, the PINGH network might consider a strategy for developing the necessary capabilities for a rotating leadership team. With a rotating system, institutions will be able to not only take the lead in guiding the organization but also take a pivotal role in guiding conversations and agendas that foster a diverse set of global health partnerships and research.

References

Belcheir MJ (2000) The National Survey of Student Engagement: results from Boise State freshmen and seniors. (Report No. BSU-RR-2000-04). Office of Institutional Advancement (ERIC Document Reproduction Service No. ED480914), Boise

Bridges BK, Kuh GD, O'Day P (2001) The National Survey of Student Engagement. https://www.naspa.org/. Accessed 27 Nov 2017

Deakin Crick R, Goldspink C (2014) Learner dispositions, self-theories and student engagement. Br J Educ Stud 62(1):19–35. https://doi.org/10.1080/00071005.2014.904038

Kuh GD (2007) What student engagement data tell us about college readiness. Peer Rev 9(1):4

Nelson Laird TF, Bridges BK, Morelon-Quainoo CL et al (2004) African American and Hispanic student engagement at minority serving and predominantly white institutions. J Coll Stud Dev 48(1):39–56. https://doi.org/10.1353/csd.2007.0005

Chapter 9
Reflections: Partnership and Collaboration in Global Health – Valuing Reciprocity

Collins O. Airhihenbuwa

In 2014, I led a team to organize the inaugural network for global health at the Pennsylvania State University (PSU) to which several institutions were invited. The inaugural network meeting built on my work for several years in which we showed that global health goals could be achieved but for it to be sustainable, partnership must be the key. Commitment alone on my part was not enough, however. There needed to be institutional support from key leaders at the university. The credit for the primary institutional champions goes to Dr. Michael Adewumi. As the vice provost for global engagement at PSU, it was Michael's vision that created a PSU global engagement network (GEN) with strategic partner institutions in different regions. The initial invitations to the inaugural network for global health were sent to the GEN institutional partners to participate in a 2-day meeting during which the global health network was launched.

Well-deserved credit also goes to Dr. Nan Crouter who as the Dean of the College of Health and Human Development supported my plan to not only host this event but also for the college to be the academic unit host for the new network. With the support of an incredible team of staff (Jodi Heaton as my assistant and Nathan Jones and the web master) we launched the network with 13 universities represented, including 3 from the US – NYU, Minnesota and Michigan. Following the inaugural meeting, Professor Neil Sharkey, as vice president for research, provided 50% of the initial funds that was matched by both Crouter and Adewumi which allowed the network to fund pilot projects over 2 years. I would like to reiterate that it took committed leaders at PSU to launch the network; institutional commitment is critical to initiating and sustaining a network such as this one. As a network, my vision was to challenge us to draw on lessons from commerce and trade in reframing spaces for engagement in partnership. For example, how do we ensure that the

C. O. Airhihenbuwa (✉)
U-Rise, St. Louis, MI, USA
e-mail: collins@u-rise.com

M. S. Winchester et al. (eds.), *Global Health Collaboration*, SpringerBriefs in Public Health, https://doi.org/10.1007/978-3-319-77685-9_9

partnership would not simply reproduce the old model of drawing raw materials from the global south, in the forms of data collection, only to be refined in the west in the form of publications with no reciprocity in production of raw materials and refinement.

As we continue to face major challenges in reducing the inequity gaps in global health, I remained committed to the vision that it is only through partnership and collaboration that we can achieve impact that are meaningful and sustainable based on the principle of reciprocity. Scholars and educators should come together with a commitment and the belief that globalization means every local space is a global space. Urbanization and the intersection of infectious and communicable diseases were the two priorities agreed to at the inaugural meeting for the network. This means that these two issues are researchable for raw materials and refinement in the global north and south. Urbanization is a major issue in Johannesburg, New York City, and Delhi and lessons from one location can inform how we address the other locations even though cultural and economic contexts may be different. The other important aspects of global health is seeking ways to bring scholars together to share knowledge and expertise rather than being fractured into the disciplines or specialization that marked one's training. It is not unusual to hear at global meetings that one group is comprised of infectious disease experts while another group, chronic disease. Yet our communities are not broken down into one or the other but instead have to confront the co-existence of these and other conditions in the same family and in some cases in the same person. I have often cited HIV/AIDS, TB and some cancers as both infectious and chronic so we are better served to examine the intersection of infectious and chronic diseases.

What Should be our Focus for the Future?
As the network and institutions evolve, it is important to examine its relevance and make adjustments to reflect changes that are likely to maximize and strengthen partnership. To that extent, I very much welcome and commend the leadership of the network for substituting 'Institution' for 'University' such that non-university institutions can find a home in the network. Such periodic reexamination is a part of the life line for any institution and network. The priority set for this network continues to be an example of where the focus should be for the future. The idea to have no more than two foci was deliberate. There are several other networks around the world and it is important that a new network has a focus and recognize that it cannot respond to all issues. Diseases intersections and urbanization are two priorities that very much align with future global direction. At the end of a meeting hosted by World Health Organization in Shanghai, China in November 2016, four key priorities were identified as the focus for health promotion globally – governance, healthy city, health literacy and social mobilization. With good governance as an overarching priority, echoing the core value of partnership in a network, healthy city and urbanization are very much aligned. Some degree of professional mobilization is called for if a network is to achieve its goals and a level of health literacy is required for us all (donors and researchers alike) to appreciate and value the important of focusing at the intersections of conditions rather than focusing on the

binaries that separate us. In the final analysis, the most important role of a network is to remind us all that it takes a collective body to have a sustainable outcome and impact on population health.

Erratum to: Provider Workload and Multiple Morbidities in the Caribbean and South Africa

Bilikisu R. Elewonibi, Shalini Pooransingh, Natalie Greaves, Linda Skaal, Tolu Oni, Madhuvanti M. Murphy, T. Alafia Samuels, and Rhonda BeLue

Erratum to:
Chapter 5 in: M. S. Winchester et al. (eds.), *Global Health Collaboration*, SpringerBriefs in Public Health, https://doi.org/10.1007/978-3-319-77685-9_5

Owing to an oversight, the names and affiliations of some of the contributing authors of this chapter were presented incorrectly. The same has been corrected throughout the book.

The updated online version of this chapter can be found at
https://doi.org/10.1007/978-3-319-77685-9_5

© The Author(s) 2018
M. S. Winchester et al. (eds.), *Global Health Collaboration*, SpringerBriefs
in Public Health, https://doi.org/10.1007/978-3-319-77685-9_10

Index